"Valerie DeLaune clearly explair ____ ____ ___ terms, what every person should know about conservative self-trea____ and the prevention of lower extremity pain. Although the author points out that trigger point therapy is often classified as alternative medicine, these proven techniques are supported by current research and based on many years of effective clinical experience. The beauty of trigger point therapy is that the average person can quickly learn the self-care techniques and incorporate them into a daily routine, measuring their own success by their steady and sometimes drastic reduction of pain and their ability to return to normal activities. If myofascial trigger points are the source of your lower extremity pain, then you will find this basic book to be a critical tool in your journey to self-healing."

—Renee Gladieux Principe, NCTMB, massage therapist and vice president of sales for the Pressure Positive Company

"There are few self-help books I can routinely recommend because most of them either dumb it down, or demand too much prior knowledge. This book is a sterling exception. I have been using trigger point therapy routinely for well over thirty years, and there was new material that rocked my boat. At the same time, the uninitiated can benefit from this book. DeLaune has synthesized a wonderful book that works as a standalone breakdown of trigger point therapy of the lower extremities or as part of her series. Any time people increase their knowledge of how to care for their bodies and start taking more responsibility, they achieve a greater level of control. This translates into a higher quality of life. Read, enjoy, and, most of all, apply!"

—Steven Lavitan, DC, chiropractor, licensed acupuncturist, and nutritionist

Trigger Point Therapy for Foot, Ankle, Knee & Leg Pain

A SELF-TREATMENT WORKBOOK

Valerie DeLaune, L.Ac.

New Harbinger Publications, Inc.

Distributed in Canada by Raincoast Books

Copyright © 2010 by Valerie DeLaune
       New Harbinger Publications, Inc.
       5674 Shattuck Avenue
       Oakland, CA 94609
       www.newharbinger.com

Cover design by Amy Shoup
Text design by Michele Waters-Kermes
Acquired by Jess O'Brien
Edited by Jean M. Blomquist

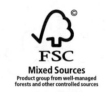

FSC
Mixed Sources
Product group from well-managed
forests and other controlled sources

Cert no. SW-COC-002283
www.fsc.org
© 1996 Forest Stewardship Council

Library of Congress Cataloging-in-Publication Data

DeLaune, Valerie.
  Trigger point therapy for foot, ankle, knee, and leg pain : a self-treatment workbook / Valerie DeLaune.
    p. cm.
  Includes bibliographical references and index.
  ISBN 978-1-57224-842-7
  1. Foot--Diseases--Chiropractic treatment--Handbooks, manuals, etc. 2. Ankle--Diseases--Chiropractic treatment--Handbooks, manuals, etc. 3. Knee--Diseases--Chiropractic treatment--Handbooks, manuals, etc. 4. Leg--Diseases--Chiropractic treatment--Handbooks, manuals, etc. 5. Pain--Alternative treatment--Handbooks, manuals, etc. 6. Self-care, Health--Handbooks, manuals, etc. I. Title.
  RZ265.F66D45 2010
  617.5'85--dc22

                      2010020701

12   11   10

10 9 8 7 6 5 4 3 2 1

First printing

Contents

Acknowledgments

Approximately 38 percent of the human population is in pain at any given time. Although 30 percent of patients seen in a general physician's practice are there due to pain caused by trigger points (Simons 2003), there is still very little emphasis in medical school on muscle pain and trigger points. Thankfully, a few pioneers have worked endlessly to research trigger points, document referral patterns and other symptoms, and bring all of that information to medical practitioners and the general public.

This book would not have been possible without the lifework of Dr. Janet Travell and Dr. David Simons, and my neuromuscular therapy instructor, Jeanne Aland, who introduced me to the books written by Doctors Travell and Simons. All three have now passed on, but I know that I and all of my patients are eternally grateful for their hard work and dedication. Their work lives on through the hundreds of thousands of patients who have gotten relief because of their research and willingness to train others.

Dr. Janet Travell

Dr. Travell was born in 1901 and followed in her father's footsteps to become a doctor. She initially specialized in cardiology but soon became interested in pain relief, as had her father. She joined her father's practice, taught at Cornell University Medical College, and pioneered and researched new pain treatments, including trigger point injections. In her private practice, she began treating Senator John F. Kennedy, who at the time was using crutches due to crippling back pain and was almost unable to walk down just a few stairs.

This was at a time when television was just beginning to bring images of politicians into the nation's living rooms, and it had become important for presidential candidates to appear physically fit. Being on crutches probably would have cost President Kennedy the election.

Dr. Travell became the first female White House physician, and after President Kennedy died, she stayed on to treat President Johnson. She resigned a year and a half later to return to her passions: teaching, lecturing, and writing about chronic myofascial pain. She continued to work into her nineties and died at the age of ninety-five on August 1, 1997.

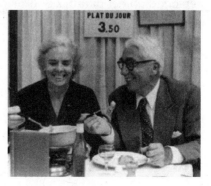

Dr. David G. Simons

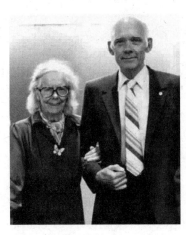

Dr. Simons, who started out his career as an aerospace physician, met Dr. Travell when she lectured at the School of Aerospace Medicine at Brooks Air Force Base in Texas in the 1960s. He soon teamed up with Dr. Travell and began researching the international literature for any references to the treatment of pain. He discovered there were a few others out there who were also discovering trigger points but using different terminology. He studied and documented the physiology of trigger points in both laboratory and clinical settings and tried to find scientific explanations for trigger points. Together Doctors Travell and Simons produced a comprehensive two-volume text on the causes and treatment of trigger points, written for physicians. Dr. Simons continued to research the physiology of trigger points, update the trigger point volumes he coauthored with Dr. Travell, and review trigger point research articles until his death at the age of 87 on April 5, 2010. He was also on the scientific advisory committee of the David G. Simons Academy, which has the goal of internationally promoting the understanding and knowledge of myofascial pain syndrome and trigger point therapy.

Other Thanks

Many additional researchers have contributed to the study of trigger points, and many doctors and other practitioners have taken the time to learn about trigger points and give that information to their patients. I would like to acknowledge all of them for their role in alleviating pain by making this important information available.

My editors Jess Beebe, Jess O'Brien, and Jean Blomquist did an excellent job providing organizational suggestions and inspiring me to make each revision even better. I would also like to thank Art Sutch, Skip Gray, and Jaime Clapp for the still photography; David Ham for being the model in the referral pattern photos; and Sarah Olsen for graphic design work. Virginia Street (Janet Travell's daughter) and Dr. Simons provided some of the photos.

I owe many thanks to the thousands of patients and some practitioners who shared with me what worked for them so that I could share that information with you. And once again, I would like to thank Sasha the dog, who was forced to wait for me while I worked too many hours to finish this book, albeit a little less patiently this time. She has learned to perfect the "stare through the window" that would force even the strongest person to do her bidding. She keeps me honest in following my own self-help techniques of taking breaks and walking for exercise.

Introduction

If you've picked up this book, chances are that you suffer from lower leg, knee, ankle, or foot pain that occurs frequently or that is intense or debilitating. You need to know that there's seldom a "magic bullet" for curing pain. In part, this is because the causes of pain are often wide-ranging and complex. Until the underlying or perpetuating factors are addressed, pain usually recurs. Lower leg, knee, ankle, or foot pain can be an intractable problem because some of the causes are seldom recognized.

What Your Health Care Provider May Not Know

The most important thing to know about trigger points is that they "refer" pain to other areas in fairly consistent patterns. For example, pain felt on the outside of your upper leg may be coming from a muscle in that area (the vastus lateralis), but it may also be coming from a trigger point located in a muscle higher up (the gluteus minimus). Knowledge of referral patterns gives us a starting point of where to look for the trigger points that are actually causing the pain.

Without a knowledge base of trigger points and referred pain, a health care provider cannot effectively treat pain syndromes. Although trigger points and their referral patterns have been documented for decades and those of us with clinical experience in trigger points have never had any doubt that they are real, only more recently have scientific double-blind controlled placebo experiments been able to "confirm" their existence (Shah et al. 2008; Chen et al. 2007). This confirmation allows the subject of trigger points to get more press in scientific and medical journals, but word is still slow in getting out to health care providers.

I've treated hundreds of fairly simple cases where people had been told their only recourse was to learn to live with their pain. The reason? Their doctor or other provider didn't know about trigger points or was unwilling to refer to an "alternative" practitioner. Thankfully, that's changing. New doctors are exposed to a wider range of alternative treatments in medical school, and some doctors who have practiced medicine for years are getting excited about exploring other treatment options.

I'm frequently contacted by people who are pretty sure trigger point treatment is at least part of the solution to their pain problems, but they are completely frustrated because they can't find a practitioner who knows about trigger points. As of this writing, massage therapists, physical therapists, and physiotherapists are the professionals who are most likely to have experience in treating trigger points. However, even if they do know about trigger points, they may not have learned much about perpetuating factors—the things that cause and keep trigger points activated and that absolutely need to be resolved for long-term relief. This is something I believe is sorely lacking in most trigger point training.

That's why learning about trigger points yourself and doing the self-help exercises in this book is so important; with the information in this book, you may be better equipped to treat trigger points than your health care provider. If you can't find someone who already knows about trigger points, bring this book to your appointments with you. Educate your practitioner about trigger points and your referral patterns. Consumer demand does drive health care, contrary to what a lot of people might think. I've seen this over the past ten years with health insurance companies; they are far more likely to cover acupuncture, massage therapy, and manual therapy (such as trigger point therapy, myofascial release, Rolfing, and related types of medical bodywork) than previously, and that's because consumers insisted on it. Health insurance companies are also finally realizing that letting consumers use lower-cost treatments saves them money in the long run.

My Background

I attended massage school in 1989 and learned Swedish massage. I learned to give a very good general massage, but trying to solve a patient's muscular problems was often frustrating and elusive. I saw a class on neuromuscular therapy (which combines a type of deep tissue massage called myofascial release with treating trigger points) in the Heartwood Institute catalog and was intrigued by the description. I attended Jeanne Aland's class in 1991, and it completely changed my approach to treating patients. Once I learned about referral patterns, I was able to start solving problems consistently, even in cases where people had been led to believe they would have to live with their pain.

Over my years of treating thousands of patients, I have added my own observations to those of Doctors Travell and Simons, and have developed a variety of self-help techniques. In 1999, I received my master's degree in acupuncture, and since then I've been specializing in treating pain syndromes and trigger points with acupuncture.

How This Book Is Organized

As you read through the book, you'll learn how muscular problems can play a very significant role in leg, knee, ankle, or foot pain, even when arthritis, mechanical injuries, and other nonmuscular conditions were the initial instigator of pain and structural damage. Because trigger points are so often involved in pain, learning self-treatment techniques is critical to obtaining long-term relief.

Part I offers background information on trigger points and why it's important to treat pain as soon as possible, including updates on what's new in trigger point research. The discovery of central sensitization and how it spreads pain to other parts of the body is very important to understanding and treating pain syndromes. Part I also describes the various causes of leg, knee, ankle, or foot pain and their relationship to trigger points, and how obesity and diabetes can compound lower extremity problems.

Part II begins the self-help sections of this book. It will help you identify the factors that are pertinent to your particular set of circumstances and symptoms, and will give suggestions you can take to help resolve them. Many things cause trigger points and keep them activated: foot *pronation* (your ankle rolls too far inward and downward with each step) and *supination* (your foot and ankle roll excessively outward), poorly designed shoes, chronic reinjuries, chronic and acute illness, emotional factors, and poor diet, to name a few. These perpetuating factors will have to be addressed in conjunction with the self-help pressure and stretching techniques in part III in order to resolve your leg, knee, ankle, or foot pain.

Part III provides instructions for locating the muscles that potentially contain trigger points, applying pressure to those trigger points, and stretching the muscles. Chapter 7 describes treatment guidelines in detail, and chapter 8 provides a guide indicating which muscle chapters you will want to consider as potential contributors to your leg, knee, ankle, or foot pain. Chapters 9 through 23 help you identify the specific muscles that are causing your pain. They contain lists of common symptoms for specific trigger points, offer helpful hints for resolving perpetuating factors for those trigger points, and describe self-treatment techniques and stretches.

How to Use This Book

Reading parts I and II will provide you with a foundation for the pressure techniques and stretches that you will learn in part III. Then, as you begin to do the pressure techniques and stretches in part III, you may find it helpful to return to parts I and II. Part II on perpetuating factors may be especially helpful because, in all likelihood, a combination of these perpetuating factors is involved in your pain. You won't get lasting relief from your trigger points (and therefore from your pain) until you address the things that are causing and aggravating your trigger points.

This is not a quick fix! There is no such thing as resolving your chronic pain in fifteen minutes or less or being pain free in five easy steps. No technique or practitioner can do that for you. I recommend that, if possible, you have your trigger points identified by a practitioner who has been trained in treating trigger points, such as a neuromuscular massage therapist or a physical therapist, and use the book to supplement their work. In my experience, people who do self-treatments at home in addition to receiving professional treatments weekly improve at least five times faster than those who receive only professional treatments.

Unfortunately, as I mentioned above, you may not have the option of locating a professional to help you. It could take longer for you to locate trigger points without the guidance of a professional, but with this book, you will most likely be able to locate the trigger points yourself. You will need to read the chapters, search for trigger points in your muscles, and use the self-treatment techniques on a regular basis until your pain is resolved. Ask yourself, "Is it worth some of my time to resolve my pain?" If the answer is yes, then you will find the information in this book very helpful.

Be sure to set realistic goals. Focus on a few muscles at a time unless there is a reason that you need to work on several together. Setting unrealistic goals can discourage you and cause you to give up. It's better to pick just a few things and do them well rather than rush through a greater number of self-help techniques or suggestions and do them poorly. You probably won't be able to apply pressure on five different muscles and stretch them, get orthotics and replace poor shoes, change your diet, and start walking every day all in the first week. Pace yourself so that this is an enjoyable process, and work on the perpetuating factors over time.

If you're working with a practitioner, they should be able to help you prioritize what needs to be done in the order of importance. If your practitioner is giving you too many things to do at once, be sure to tell them that you are overwhelmed and need to set priorities. Giving a patient too many assignments is all too easy for a practitioner to do, especially when they are first out of school and brimming with many useful ideas and suggestions.

There are hundreds of suggestions in this book. As you read through part II on perpetuating factors and the "Helpful Hints" in chapters about the muscles you have identified as potentially causing your pain referral patterns, highlight anything that might be pertinent to your situation. Then plan to devote some time to accomplishing your goals. Resolving pain is like detective work—what causes your pain and also what resolves it will be a combination of factors unique to you. This book gives you numerous tools for your process of self-discovery on the road to relief from pain.

Part I

TRIGGER POINTS & FOOT, ANKLE, KNEE, AND LOWER LEG PAIN

If you're suffering from leg, knee, ankle, or foot pain, all too often you may be diagnosed with general terms such as arthritis, tendinitis, plantar fasciitis, or shin splints without the true cause being identified. Often the cause is trigger points in one or more muscles, but the diagnosing practitioner is unfamiliar with trigger points. Trigger points can play a very large role in most pain syndromes, which means that you may be able to get a great deal of relief, or even complete relief, by working on trigger points and eliminating perpetuating factors.

The sooner you start doing the self-help techniques and possibly receiving treatment from a practitioner, the sooner you will feel better. This is important, since untreated pain can create an escalating cycle that makes it more chronic and more resistant to treatment.

Chapter 1

What Are Trigger Points?

In this chapter, you'll learn what trigger points are, how they form, and what it feels like when they're pressed. You'll also learn how they refer pain to areas of the body remote from the trigger point itself, what symptoms they can cause besides pain, and what happens when they're left untreated.

Characteristics of Trigger Points

Muscle is the largest organ in the human body, typically accounting for almost 50 percent of the body's weight. There are approximately four hundred muscles in the human body (surprisingly, there are individual variations), and any one of them can develop trigger points, potentially causing referred pain and dysfunction. Symptoms can range from intolerable, agonizing pain to painless restriction of movement and distorted posture.

Knots, Tight Bands, and Tenderness in the Muscle

Muscles consist of many muscle cells, or fibers, bundled together and surrounded by connective tissue. Each fiber contains numerous myofibrils, and most skeletal muscles contain approximately one thousand to two thousand myofibrils. Each myofibril consists of a chain of sarcomeres connected end-to-end. Muscular contractions take place in the sarcomere. When a trigger point is present, numerous sarcomeres are contracted into a small, thickened area and the rest of the sarcomeres in the myofibril are stretched thin. Several of these contractures in the same area are probably what we feel as a "knot" or "tight band" in the muscle. These muscle fibers are not available for use because they are already contracted, which is why you cannot condition (strengthen) a muscle that contains trigger points.

When pressed, trigger points are usually very tender. The sustained contraction of the fibril leads to the release of sensitizing *neurochemicals* (body substances that affect the nervous system), producing the pain that is felt when the trigger point is pressed. Pain intensity levels can vary depending on the amount of stress placed on the muscles. The intensity of pain can also vary in response to flare-ups of any of the perpetuating factors addressed in part II, including emotional factors, illnesses, and insomnia.

Healthy muscles usually do not contain knots or tight bands, are not tender to pressure, and, when not in use, feel soft and pliable to the touch, not like the hard and dense muscles found in people with chronic pain. People often tell me their muscles feel hard and dense because they work out and do strengthening exercises, but healthy muscles feel soft and pliable when not being used, even if you work out.

Referred Pain

Trigger points may refer pain in the local area and/or to other areas of the body, and the most common patterns have been well documented and diagramed. These are called *referral patterns*. Approximately half of the time, trigger points are not located in the same place where you feel symptoms. In part III, you'll find illustrations of common pain referral patterns that you can compare with your pain patterns, and this will help you figure out where the trigger point or points causing your pain are located. If you don't know that you need to search those locations and, instead, you work only on the areas where you feel pain, you probably won't get relief. For example, trigger points in the soleus muscle (part of your calf) can cause pain over the back of the knee, down the calf, and into the heel and bottom of the foot, and then the heel pain frequently gets misdiagnosed as plantar fasciitis.

If you have been in pain for a long time, *central sensitization* (discussed below) can cause the pain referral to deviate from the most commonly found pattern. It may also cause trigger points in several muscles in a region to all refer pain to one area, making it all the harder to determine the actual source of the referred pain. This means you can't absolutely rule out the role of a potential trigger point based only on consideration of common referral patterns, since other factors may cause you to have an *uncommon* referral pattern. The more intense the earlier pain, the more intense the emotions associated with it, and the longer it has gone on, the more likely central sensitization will cause deviation from the most common referral patterns (Simons, Travell, and Simons 1999).

When you apply pressure to the trigger point, you can often reproduce the referred pain or other symptoms, but being unable to reproduce the referred pain or other symptoms by applying pressure does not rule out involvement of that specific trigger point. Try treating the trigger points that could be causing the problem anyway, and if you improve, even temporarily, assume that one of the trigger points you worked on is indeed at least part of the problem. For this reason, don't work on all the possible trigger points in one session, since you won't know which trigger point treated actually gave you relief.

Referred tingling, numbness, or burning sensations are more likely due to trigger points constricting around or putting pressure on a nerve. For example, the sciatic nerve runs either under or through the piriformis muscle in the gluteal area, and trigger points in the piriformis muscle can compress the sciatic nerve, causing a pseudosciatic pain that runs down the back of the leg and mimics true sciatica, which is caused by compression of the lumbar spine nerve roots from ruptured discs or bone spurs.

Weakness and Muscle Fatigue

Trigger points cause weakness and loss of coordination of the involved muscles, along with an inability of the muscles to tolerate use. Many people take this as a sign that they need to strengthen the weak muscles, but if the trigger points aren't inactivated first, strengthening (conditioning) exercises will likely encourage the surrounding muscles to do the work instead of the muscle containing the trigger point, further weakening and deconditioning the muscle containing trigger points.

Muscles containing trigger points are fatigued more easily and don't return to a relaxed state as quickly when use of the muscle ceases. In addition, trigger points may cause other muscles to tighten up and become weak and fatigued in the areas where you experience the referred pain, and also cause a generalized tightening of an area as a response to pain.

Other Symptoms

Trigger points can cause symptoms not normally associated with muscular problems. For example, trigger points in the vastus medialis muscle, in addition to causing pain in the knee, can also cause the knee to buckle unexpectedly, while trigger points in the vastus lateralis, in addition to causing pain over the outside of the thigh, can cause the kneecap to lock so that you can't bend your leg.

You may suffer from stiff joints, fatigue, generalized weakness, twitching, trembling, and areas of numbness or other odd sensations. It probably wouldn't occur to you (or your health care practitioner) that these symptoms could be caused by a trigger point in a muscle.

Active Phase vs. Latent Phase

A trigger point can be in either an active or a latent phase, depending on how irritated it is. If the trigger point is *active,* it will refer pain or other sensations and limit range of motion. If the trigger point is *latent,* it may cause only a decreased range of motion and weakness, but not pain. The more frequent and intense your pain, the greater the number of active trigger points you're likely to have.

Trigger points that start with some impact to the muscle, such as an injury, are usually active initially. Poor posture or poor body mechanics, repetitive use, a nerve root irritation, or any of the other perpetuating factors addressed in part II can also form active trigger points. Active trigger points may at some point stop referring pain and become latent. However, these latent trigger points can easily become active again, which may lead you to believe you're experiencing a new problem when in fact an old problem—perhaps even something you've forgotten about—is being reaggravated.

Latent trigger points can be reactivated by overuse, overstretching, or muscle chilling. Any of the perpetuating factors discussed in part II can activate previously latent trigger points and make you more prone to developing new trigger points initiated by impacts to muscles. Latent trigger points can also develop gradually without being active first, and you don't even know they are there. In a study of thirteen healthy people with the same eight muscles examined in each (Simons

2003), two people had latent trigger points in seven of those muscles, one person had latent trigger points in six muscles, three had latent trigger points in five muscles, two had latent trigger points in three muscles, two had latent trigger points in two muscles, two had latent trigger points in one muscle, and only one person didn't have latent trigger points in any of the eight muscles! This means that most people have at least some latent trigger points, which can easily be converted to active trigger points. This also means that some people are more prone to developing problems with muscular pain than others.

Primary and Satellite Trigger Points

A *primary*, or *key*, trigger point can cause a *satellite*, or *secondary*, trigger point to develop in a different muscle. The latter may form because it lies within the referral zone of the primary trigger point. Alternatively, the muscle with the satellite trigger point may be overloaded because it's substituting for the muscle with the primary trigger point, or it may be countering the tension in the muscle with the primary trigger point. When doing self-treatments, be aware that some of your trigger points may be satellite trigger points, in which case you won't be able to treat them effectively until the primary trigger points causing them have been treated. Part III offers guidance in this regard.

Elevated Biochemicals

A ground-breaking 2008 study (Shah et al.) was able to measure eleven elevated biochemicals in and surrounding active trigger points, including inflammatory mediators, neuropeptides, catecholamines, and cytokines (primarily sensitizing substances and immune system biochemicals). In addition, the pH of the samples was strongly acidic compared to other areas of the body. A 1996 study by Issbener, Reeh, and Steen found that a localized acidic pH lowers the pain threshold sensitivity level of sensory receptors (part of the nervous system), even without acute damage to the muscle. This means the more acidic your pH level in a given area, the more easily you will experience pain compared to someone else. Further studies are needed to discover whether body-wide elevations in pH acidity and the substances mentioned above predispose people to develop trigger points.

What Happens When You Leave Trigger Points Untreated?

When people first develop some kind of pain problem, they usually wait to see if it will go away. Sometimes it does, and sometimes it doesn't. The problem with "waiting to see" is that when trigger points are left untreated, muscles can be damaged, and eventually changes to the central nervous system can lead to a vicious cycle of pain. This central nervous system involvement probably explains why you are experiencing chronic pain.

Damage to the Muscle Fibers

Remember how trigger points cause portions of the myofibril to stay contracted? If this goes on too long, the myofibril may break in the middle, causing it to retract to each end and leave an empty shell in the middle. Muscle fibers damaged in this way cannot be repaired and will never be available for use again (Simons, Travell, and Simons 1999).

Central Nervous System Sensitization

The purpose of the acute stress responses of our bodies is to protect us and let us know we need to change something in our lives, whether it is pulling away from a hot stove burner, fleeing from a dangerous situation, or giving an injured body part time to heal. But when emotional and/or physical stress (including pain) is prolonged, even just for days, there is a maladaptive response: damage to the central nervous system, particularly to the sympathetic nervous system and the hypothalamus-pituitary-adrenal (HPA) system. This is called central sensitization.

Certain types of nerve receptors in muscles relay information to neurons located within part of the gray matter of the spinal cord and the brain stem. Pain is amplified there and then is relayed to other muscle areas, thereby expanding the region of pain beyond the initially affected area. Once the central nervous system is involved, or *sensitized* in this way, persistent pain leads to long-term or permanent changes in these neurons, which affect adjacent neurons through *neurotransmitters* (chemical substances that are produced and secreted by a neuron and then diffuse across *synapses*, or small gaps, between neurons, causing excitation or inhibition of another neuron). This may also cause the part of the nervous system that would normally counteract pain to malfunction and fail to do its job (Borg-Stein and Simons 2002; Niddam 2009; Latremoliere and Woolf 2009). As a result, pain can be more easily triggered by lower levels of physical and emotional stressors, and also can be more intense and last longer. Conditions of chronic inflammation, such as osteoarthritis and rheumatoid arthritis, also cause central nervous system sensitization, leading to a vicious cycle of pain.

And while prolonged exposure to both emotional and physical stressors can lead to central nervous system sensitization and subsequently cause pain, prolonged pain caused by central nervous system sensitization can lead to emotional and physical stress (Niddam 2009). Just the central nervous system maladaptive changes alone can be self-perpetuating and cause pain, even without the presence of either the original or any additional stressors (Latremoliere and Woolf 2009).

So the longer pain goes untreated, the greater the number of neurons that get involved and the more muscles they affect, causing pain in new areas, in turn causing more neurons to get involved—and the bigger the problem becomes, leading to the likelihood that the pain will become a chronic problem. The sooner pain is treated, including addressing the initiating stressors and perpetuating factors, the less likely it will become a permanent problem with widespread muscle involvement and central nervous system changes.

Sensitization of the Opposite Side of the Body

You may be surprised to discover that the same area on the opposite side of your body is also tender to pressure, even though that side isn't otherwise painful. Over half of the time, the opposite side is actually more tender with pressure. Unless it is a recent injury, it's typical for both sides to eventually get involved (for example, if the right calf is painful, there are likely to be tender points in the left calf). Whatever is affecting one leg is likely affecting the other, whether it's directly from poor body mechanics, poor footwear, or overuse injuries, or indirectly from chronic degenerative or inflammatory conditions, chronic disease, and central sensitization. For that reason, I almost always work on both sides, and I recommend that you do self-treatments on both sides.

This observation has been supported by a study in which the researchers used needle electrodes placed in the same spot on both sides of the neck or back to record muscle electrical activity (Audette, Wang, and Smith 2004). When an active trigger point was stimulated on one side of the body, it induced electrical muscle activity on the corresponding opposite side. Latent trigger points did not produce the same results. This further supports the concept of central nervous system sensitization, which would cause corresponding trigger points to form on the opposite side of the body over time.

How Trigger Points Form

Trigger points may form after a sudden trauma or injury, or they may develop gradually. Common initiating and perpetuating factors are mechanical stresses, injuries, nutritional problems, emotional factors, sleep problems, acute or chronic infections, organ dysfunction and disease, and other medical conditions. Part II goes into detail about these causes and perpetuators of trigger points.

Part of the current hypothesis about the mechanism responsible for the formation of trigger points is the *energy crisis component theory*. The *sarcoplasmic reticulum*, a part of each cell, is responsible for storing and releasing ionized calcium. The type of nerve ending that causes the muscle fiber to contract is called a *motor end plate*. This nerve ending releases *acetylcholine*, a neurotransmitter that tells the sarcoplasmic reticulum to release calcium, and then the muscle fiber contracts. If it is operating normally, when contraction of the muscle fiber is no longer needed, the nerve ending stops releasing acetylcholine, and the calcium pump in the sarcoplasmic reticulum returns calcium into the sarcoplasmic reticulum. If a trauma occurs or there is a large increase in the motor end plate's release of acetylcholine, an excessive amount of calcium can be released by the sarcoplasmic reticulum, causing a maximal contracture of a segment of muscle, leading to a maximal demand for energy and impairment of local circulation. If circulation is impeded, the calcium pump doesn't get the fuel and oxygen it needs to pump calcium back into the sarcoplasmic reticulum, so the muscle fiber continues to contract.

The areas at the ends of the muscle fibers (either at the bone or where the muscle attaches to a tendon) also become tender as the attachments are stressed by the contraction in the center of the fiber (Simons, Travell, and Simons 1999). Once the central nervous system has been sensitized, various substances are released: *histamine* (a compound that causes dilation and permeability of blood vessels), *serotonin* (a neurotransmitter that constricts blood vessels), *bradykinin* (a hormone that dilates peripheral blood vessels and increases small blood vessel permeability), and *substance P* (a compound involved in the regulation of the pain threshold). These substances stimulate the nervous system to release even more acetylcholine locally, adding to the perpetuation of the dysfunctional cycle (Borg-Stein and Simons 2002). This vicious cycle continues until some sort of outside intervention stretches the contracted portion of the muscle fiber. Anxiety and nervous tension also increase *autonomic nervous system* activity (the part of the nervous system that controls the release of acetylcholine, along with involuntary functions of blood vessels and glands), which commonly aggravates trigger points and their associated symptoms (Simons 2004). Studies by Partanen, Ojala, and Arokoski (2009), Shah et al. (2008), and Kuan (2009) support Simon's hypothesis.

Conclusion

Trigger points are tender when pressed, and the multiple contractures forming the trigger point may feel like a small lump in the muscle. Healthy muscles don't contain trigger points, and they don't feel tender with pressure. If trigger points are left untreated, the damage to the muscle cells can be irreparable and will cause long-term changes in the central nervous system, leading to a self-perpetuating cycle of trigger points, pain, and muscular damage. Trigger points can cause symptoms other than pain, which should be taken into consideration and may help you determine which muscles contain trigger points. This is particularly important when the referral pattern deviates from the common pattern, making the location of the trigger points harder to determine.

In the next chapter, you'll learn more about treating trigger points and when you should see a doctor.

Chapter 2

You Don't Need to Live with Pain

It is important to treat trigger points as soon as possible so that they are less likely to cause chronic pain problems. This chapter explains the importance of prompt treatment, and also gives you some idea of what to expect from treatment and when you might need to consult a health care provider. Part III outlines general guidelines for self-treatment and teaches you how to treat the trigger points involved in leg, knee, ankle, or foot pain.

Pain Is Treatable

People often assume that if a parent had the same type of condition, it must be genetic and they'll just have to learn to live with it. I never operate on the assumption that a condition can't be improved, even if it is genetic. You learn many things from your parents—eating habits, exercise habits, how to deal with stressful situations, even posture and gestures—and all of these things can influence your own health.

I never assume I can't help someone, or that I can't think of someone to refer them to, such as a chiropractor, naturopath, or surgeon who can help them. In spite of being told that you have to learn to live with your medical condition, assume you can change it—at least until you have exhausted all current treatment options.

The Importance of Prompt Treatment

So often I hear patients say, "I kept thinking it would go away." Sometimes symptoms will go away in a few days and never return. But more often, the longer you wait to see if pain will go away, the more muscles become involved in the chain reaction of chronic pain and dysfunction. A muscle hurts and forms trigger points, then the area of referral (where you feel the pain or other symptoms) starts to hurt and tighten up and forms its own satellite trigger points, then those trigger points refer pain somewhere else, and so on. Or the pain may improve for a while, but the trigger points are really just in an inactive phase and can readily become active and cause pain or other symptoms once again.

As explained in chapter 1, eventually there will be permanent structural damage to the muscle cells and sensitization of the central nervous system. The problem gets more complex the longer trigger points are left untreated, becoming more painful, more debilitating, more frustrating, and more time-consuming and expensive to treat. Plus, the longer you wait, the less likely you are to get complete relief—and the more likely it is that your trigger points will be reactivated chronically and periodically.

Breaking the Pain Cycle

Something starts to hurt, so you tense the area up. Then it hurts more, so the muscle tightens up more, perpetuating and escalating the cycle of pain. Any intervention that helps treat trigger points and eliminate perpetuating factors can help break the cycle: trigger point self-treatments, stretching, heat and/or ice, chiropractic or osteopathic treatments, massage, ultrasound, homeopathy, biofeedback, trigger point injections, counseling, and even analgesics.

People are often surprised that I support the use of analgesics, such as aspirin and ibuprofen, but anything that breaks the pain cycle as soon as possible helps prevent the symptoms from getting worse or affecting other muscles. Plus, analgesics can help you tolerate the initial stages of treatment if you are in extreme pain. But be aware that just because your pain level has decreased, this doesn't mean the trigger points are gone. You still need to seek treatment, preferably as soon as possible. Analgesics will most likely take the edge off the pain, but unless you plan to take them as a long-term solution, you also need to treat the source of the problem.

Muscle relaxants are of limited value for people with pain caused by trigger points because muscle spasms are not the cause of the pain. Also, these drugs first release tension in the muscles that provide *protective splinting* (the muscles that contract to compensate for or protect the weakened muscles containing the trigger points). Removing this protective splinting increases the load on the muscle containing trigger points and leads to additional pain.

Why Trigger Point Therapy Works

Massage and self-treatment of trigger points will allow muscle cells to take up more oxygen and nutrients and eliminate metabolic wastes again, which is the proper cell metabolism process. Also, pressing on the trigger points and making the muscle hurt a little bit more than it's already hurting causes your body to release pain-masking chemicals such as endorphins, thereby breaking the pain cycle.

How Long Will Therapy Take?

When people begin therapy, they commonly ask me, "How long will it take?" My general rule of thumb is that the longer the condition has been going on and the more medical conditions (of any kind) you have, the greater the number of muscles that will become involved through central sensitization. This means that treatment will be more complex and take longer. If you are perfectly healthy and have only a recent minor injury, you may not need long-term treatment.

Major factors in the amount of time it takes to get relief from symptoms are how diligently you perform self-treatments, and how accurately you identify your perpetuating factors (discussed in part II) and succeed in eliminating them. As I noted in the introduction, in my experience, people who do self-treatments at home in addition to receiving weekly professional treatments improve at least five times faster than those who receive only professional treatments. Doctors Travell and Simons said, "Treatments that are done *to* the patient should be minimized and effort should be concentrated in teaching what can be done *by* the patient… As patients exercise increasing control [over symptom management,] they improve both physically and emotionally" (1992, 549).

I can usually give patients a pretty good indication of how many treatments they may need by the end of the second or third treatment, based on their medical condition, how their muscles feel to me, their diligence about self-treatment and working on perpetuating factors, and how much they have improved (or not) within the first few weeks. If you are seeing a practitioner, after a few weeks ask for an assessment of how long and how frequently the practitioner expects to see you. They may be able to at least give you an idea based on what they have seen so far.

A small percentage of people will get worse before they get better, mostly in complex cases. Or the pain may move around, or you may have the perception that the pain moved around only because the worst areas have improved and now you are noticing the next-worst area more. If the self-treatments are uncomfortable, try to find ways to ease the discomfort, such as reducing the frequency of treatments or decreasing the amount of pressure. It's helpful to keep a journal or other record of your pain and other symptoms. Chapter 8 includes a page with a human body outline that you can photocopy and use to document your pain. This will help you determine whether you're making progress, even at times when you don't perceive any changes in your symptoms. Also seek feedback from people who are close to you. Often they will notice progress in your mobility and activity level, even if you aren't aware of it.

I've had only a few cases where I wasn't able to help patients, and in these cases the people were so frustrated (and understandably so) after seeing professional after professional and receiving little or no help that they allowed me to treat them only a few times before giving up, even if they had improved. If you get a little worse before you get better, you may be inclined to give up in the initial stages of treatment. I encourage you to give any treatment you try some amount of time before you decide it isn't working, even if your condition initially gets worse. Most professionals have numerous tools in their bag, and if something isn't working, they can try something else. It is not realistic to expect your practitioner to figure it all out and give you a large amount of relief within the first appointment or two. Just give your practitioner some time to learn your body and observe how you use it. However, if a practitioner doesn't seem to care or have time for you, then by all means look for someone who cares about you getting better.

When Should You See a Health Care Provider?

If you can't get relief by using the self-help techniques in this book, you will need to see a health care provider. It may be that something other than trigger points is causing or contributing to your leg, knee, ankle, or foot pain. X-rays, MRIs, and other diagnostic tests can identify some conditions that may cause pain, such as osteoarthritis, torn ligaments or tendons, and stress fractures. Referred symptoms due to trigger points can mimic other, more serious conditions or occur concurrently with them. It may take some investigation to determine the ultimate cause of the problem, which will determine how it can most effectively be treated.

You should see a doctor immediately to rule out serious conditions if you have pain in your legs and feet with any of the following symptoms:

- Your pain had a sudden onset, is severe, or starts with a traumatic injury, particularly if you heard a noise at the time or it felt as if someone had hit you with something hard.

- Your pain lasts for more than two weeks.

- The intensity of pain increases over time, or the symptoms are different (changes can be an indication of a different, more serious cause).

- Your pain is accompanied by redness, heat, severe swelling, or odd sensations, particularly over the calves.

- You develop rashes or ulcers that don't heal.

- You are experiencing chronic calf cramping.

- You develop poor circulation, painful varicose veins, and very cold legs, feet, arms, or hands.

Hopefully your doctor will rule out any serious conditions. If you are diagnosed with pain from structural damage or chronic conditions, chances are you can relieve much or all of your pain with a combination of self-treatment of trigger points and treating and eliminating the perpetuating factors. Regardless of the diagnosis you receive from a health care provider, my general treatment principle is the same: identify and eliminate all the underlying causes to the extent possible, and treat the trigger points.

Conclusion

The most important thing to learn from this chapter is that you don't necessarily have to live with your pain. There are treatment options, even if your current practitioner isn't aware of all of them. Analgesics, such as ibuprofen, and use of heat and cold can help break the pain cycle, but they are not a substitute for treatment of trigger points and elimination of perpetuating factors. The length of treatment will depend on your individual medical condition and how long the condition has been going on, and your commitment to doing self-treatments and identifying and addressing perpetuating factors. You may possibly get worse before you get better, but this shouldn't necessarily alarm you. If you have any of the symptoms listed above or the self-help techniques in this book aren't helping, see a medical provider.

The next chapter will address specific types of leg, knee, ankle, and foot pain, and the role of trigger points in causing and perpetuating associated conditions.

Chapter 3

Foot, Ankle, Knee, and Lower Leg Pain

Incidences of leg and foot pain are on a dramatic rise due to an increase in the number of acute injuries, and because of the increasing number of people with medical conditions that affect the legs. The associated medical costs are staggering (Hinkers 2009).

Acute injuries are most often due to sports injuries caused by improper training (including "weekend warrior" syndrome). If you are a sports enthusiast, properly warming up with stretches and mild exercise will go a long way toward preventing injuries. *Cross-training*, or exercises that use different muscle groups in different ways, helps by strengthening multiple muscle groups. If you participate only in one or two sports, you will strengthen only certain muscles, allowing others to be deconditioned. This sets you up for acute and chronic injuries, and also leads to the formation of trigger points.

Chronic medical conditions such as diabetes, atherosclerosis, and obesity, which are most often the result of a sedentary lifestyle combined with a poor diet, can also indirectly cause and perpetuate trigger points. Because the muscles in the legs and feet support the entire weight of the body, they can be particularly susceptible to mechanical stresses, and because they are farthest from the heart, they are more likely to suffer from the poor circulation characteristic of these medical conditions. Diabetes and obesity will be discussed in more detail in part II.

This chapter addresses the most common sources of pain from injuries and chronic conditions, and how trigger points can potentially be involved either directly or indirectly.

Knee Pain

There can be several causes of knee pain, such as osteoarthritis, problems with the kneecap alignment, inflammation of one of the lubricating sacs of fluid in the knee (true bursitis), and damage to the cartilage, tendons, and ligaments from either overuse injuries or sudden traumatic injuries. If you had a sudden impact to your knee or leg and are experiencing severe pain in the knee area, you will want to see a doctor to be evaluated for structural damage.

If you have been diagnosed with some kind of tear or rupture, surgery may be necessary to repair the damage. Trigger point self-help techniques will be valuable pre- and postsurgery to keep the muscles as relaxed as possible, to speed healing, and to help minimize the potential long-term effects of peripheral and central sensitization.

Pain that has come on gradually is more likely due to an overuse injury, an inflammatory process such as bursitis, or a degenerative condition such as osteoarthritis. Try the trigger point self-help techniques included in this book to see if you can relieve the pain. If you can't reduce or relieve your pain fairly quickly, you will want to see a health care provider for an evaluation for structural damage. No matter what the cause, you will want to continue to apply pressure to trigger points.

Remember central sensitization from chapter 1? Information from the knee joint is processed in both the superficial and deep dorsal horn of the spinal cord, and deep tissues are particularly capable of inducing central sensitization. This means that central sensitization from both osteoarthritis and inflammatory joint disease can induce pain beyond the region of the joint and eventually form trigger points in the surrounding muscles. This may be why people with joint replacements still experience pain—it could be a result of trigger point pain referral, even though trigger points were not originally part of the underlying disease.

Some of the more common problems affecting the knee are worth mentioning in more detail, especially those that can either be caused by or cause trigger points, such as osteoarthritis, patellofemoral pain, iliotibial band syndrome, tendinopathies and muscle strains, bursitis, meniscus tears, and ligament sprains and tears.

Osteoarthritis

Osteoarthritis (OA) is the most common joint disorder, and the knee is the joint most commonly affected. The cartilage cushioning the knee joint wears away first, and then, as the degeneration progresses, the underlying bone can also wear away. This degeneration process causes the ends of the bones to become thicker, and they may form *osteophytes*, or spurs. It is presently unclear at which stage in the degeneration process the joint becomes painful. While pain from OA is usually localized to the affected joint, hip OA may cause knee pain.

Symptoms may include a deep aching pain in the joint that gets worse after exercise or when putting weight on it, stiffness, limited mobility, a grating sound, joint swelling, and pain that is worse at night and with rainy weather. Resting the joint gives you relief. In the earlier stages, the pain may be episodic, but in advanced stages pain may be constant.

Risk factors are age, obesity, muscle weakness, and past injury. Women are affected more often than men. Almost half of American adults may develop osteoarthritis in at least one knee by age 85, with the likelihood increasing both with age and as body mass increases with weight problems. Sixty-six percent of obese adults will develop osteoarthritis in one or both knees (Murphy et al. 2008). Other risk factors include structural misalignment, muscle weakness, genetic predisposition, and certain professions that require hard labor, heavy lifting, knee bending, and repetitive motion. Once knee osteoarthritis degeneration starts, it becomes a vicious cycle. Your knee hurts, so you exercise less, which leads to muscle weakness and possibly to weight gain, which adds to the degeneration progression.

While advancing age and genetic predisposition are not within your control, modifying your work environment with correct ergonomic furniture and changing the way you use your body, along with changing your diet (if necessary), are things you can do fairly easily and relatively inexpensively. Structural misalignments and muscle weakness can be corrected with the help of a doctor, chiropractor, or physical therapist. You can do a lot to help stop the progression of osteo-arthritis or prevent it before it starts. Many of the self-help techniques in parts II and III of this book will be very helpful for treating trigger points that have already formed and for preventing additional trigger points from forming.

Patellofemoral Pain (Chrondromalacia Patellae)

The kneecap (patella) is a small bone with some cartilage on the side closest to the joint. The cartilage provides shock absorption and allows the kneecap to move smoothly through a groove that is formed by the ends of the lower leg and thigh bones (tibia and femur) behind the kneecap. Pain around the kneecap that develops gradually is usually caused by muscle imbalances, where the vastus lateralis and rectus femoris muscles are tight, and the vastus medialis is not conditioned. This pulls the kneecap a little toward the outside of the leg, and it no longer tracks properly in the groove. The cartilage rubs against the underlying bone and gets damaged over time. If the cartilage is damaged by an impact to the front of the kneecap, it can cause small tears or roughening of the cartilage, leading to pain.

If the cartilage has been damaged, symptoms may include a grinding or clicking when you are straightening your knee, pain that is worse when walking down stairs, pain upon standing up after sitting for a long period, possibly pain when pressing against the kneecap, and maybe slight swelling.

Muscle imbalances are usually easily solved by using the self-help techniques for trigger points found in the vastus lateralis and rectus femoris muscle chapters in part III, and by strengthening the vastus medialis muscle. If the cartilage is not damaged, you should get relief quickly. Other muscles that may need treatment are the gluteal muscles and the tensor fascia latae, which are beyond the scope of this book. Correcting for foot pronation may also help, and will be addressed in chapter 4, under "Self-help technique: Choose appropriate footwear."

If the cartilage has been damaged, surgery may be necessary, but as noted above, the techniques in this book will help you both pre- and postsurgery, and also help to realign the kneecap and prevent further damage.

Iliotibial Band Syndrome (Runner's Knee)

The iliotibial (IT) band is connective tissue that attaches to the top of your pelvis and the tensor fascia latae muscle, runs down the side of the leg, and attaches on the outside of the tibia just below the knee. If the IT band is tight, as is common in runners, it can rub across the bony prominence at the bottom of the femur on the outside of the knee.

Symptoms may include pain on the outside of your knee that is worse with running, tightness along the outside of your thigh, pain when flexing and extending your lower leg, weakness in moving your leg out away from your body, and tightness in the gluteal and tensor fascia latae muscles.

True IT band syndrome can be confused with referred pain from trigger points in the posterior portion of the gluteus minimus, the tensor fascia latae, and the vastus lateralis muscles, since referred pain from trigger points in the first two muscles is felt on the outside of the thigh, and the vastus lateralis refers pain both over the outside of the thigh and into the knee. Because this book addresses only referred pain from the knee on down and not in the thigh, self-help techniques are included only for the vastus lateralis muscle. By working on that muscle, you can likely reduce or eliminate pain from IT band syndrome, but you may want to see the Resources section at the end of this book for books that cover additional muscles.

Quadriceps Muscles and Patellar Tendinopathy

The quadriceps tendon attaches your quadriceps muscle to your kneecap, and the patellar tendon runs from your kneecap to the tibia (the larger of the two lower leg bones). If stress is placed on the tendons, they can develop tiny tears (previously known as tendinitis or tendinosis). Tendons heal more slowly than muscles because they don't have as ample a blood supply.

A variety of factors may be involved in developing tendinopathies, including sudden increases in the intensity and frequency of exercise, misalignment of your leg bones, muscular imbalances, tight thigh and other leg muscles, and being overweight. Symptoms may include an increase in pain and maybe a crunchy sound or feeling when using the tendon, and/or increased pain and stiffness at night or upon waking; the area may also be tender, red, warm, or swollen. The symptoms can easily be confused with bursitis. Treating trigger points using the methods taught in this book can relieve the tightness of muscles pulling on the tendons, prevent further damage to the tendons, reduce or stop pain, and allow the tendons to heal.

Hamstring Muscles/Tendinopathy and Strains

Tightness in the hamstring muscles can also stress and cause injuries to both the muscles and the associated tendons, for the same reasons as noted above for the quadriceps muscles. The hamstring tendons attach on the bones of the lower leg, just below the knee area.

Symptoms of tendinopathy include pain when pressure is applied over the tendon attachment, pain upon bending your knee combined with resistance pressure applied against the calf, and stiffness after exercise. Treating hamstring muscle trigger points using the methods taught in this book can relieve the tightness of muscles pulling on the tendons, prevent further damage to muscles and the tendons, reduce or stop pain, and allow the tendons to heal. If the biceps femoris tendon is completely torn (which is likely only with a rapid movement as required by certain sports), the torn area will swell. If you have swelling or severe pain, you will need to see a doctor for treatment and evaluation. Treating the tight muscles and trigger points can help prevent this kind of injury, as a relaxed muscle is less prone to injury than a tight one.

Bursitis

Though *true* bursitis may have little to do with trigger points except possibly indirectly (if the ligament or tendon from a tight muscle contributes to the friction that may be causing bursitis), I wanted to mention it because often pain in or over the joint is misdiagnosed as bursitis, when in fact it is actually referred pain from trigger points.

A *bursa* is a small, fluid-filled sac that allows skin, tendons, muscles, and ligaments to slide easily over the underlying bone. Bursa are found in and near joints such as the knee, over the trochanter of the femur bone (what most people would point to as their hip bone area), shoulder, and elbow. Bursitis of the knee can be caused by a traumatic blow to the bursa, by repeated pressure leading to irritation (such as repeated kneeling, as in the old terms "housemaid's knee" or "clergyman's knee"), and by infections. Symptoms include pain and tenderness on and just below the kneecap, pain when kneeling, and possibly swelling and warmth or even an abscess or fluid-filled lump. I believe it is worth checking for trigger points in the muscles surrounding the joint, just in case trigger points and tight muscles are causing the friction and irritating the bursa sac, or in case it is not really bursitis causing your knee pain.

Meniscus Tears

The *lateral* (outer side) and *medial* (inner side) menisci are cartilage that acts as shock absorbers for the knee. Damage can be from an acute injury or degenerative changes, and damage to the medial meniscus is more common.

Symptoms may include swelling, tenderness, or pain on the inside or outside of your knee right next to the joint. Pain is increased by bending the knee, and you may possibly hear popping, cracking, or clicking. This needs to be diagnosed by a doctor. If you had a sudden injury accompanied by a sound, you will certainly need to see a doctor for evaluation. If a tear is found, depending on the extent of the injury, the treatment may either be conservative—including icing, pain medications, ultrasound or laser therapy, massage/manual therapy, and eventually conditioning exercises—or surgery if the damage is more severe. Herbs and other supplements for healing traumatic injuries as well as acupuncture will be helpful (see page 42). With either the conservative or surgical option, self-compression of trigger points will be helpful, as long as you don't stress your joints. Do not perform stretches without the guidance of your health care practitioner. Use pain as a guideline: if it hurts, don't do it—at least until you are under the supervision of a physical therapist.

Knee Ligament Sprains and Tears

Ligaments are connective tissue that attach bone to bone. In the knee, the two cruciate ligaments and the medial collateral ligaments attach the femur to the tibia. The lateral collateral ligament attaches the femur to the head of the fibula, the thinner bone in the lower leg.

Damage is usually caused by an injury as opposed to overuse, and can lead to or be found in combination with a meniscus tear (see above) or an injury to the articular cartilage (a pad between the femur and the tibia). Symptoms can range from mild tenderness over the ligament for a mild injury, to pain and knee instability if there is a complete tear of the ligament, and possibly swelling depending on which ligament is affected and the severity of the injury. The treatments under meniscus tears also apply to knee ligament tears.

Calf Pain

There are two large muscles in the calf—the gastrocnemius and the soleus—along with some other smaller muscles. Trigger points can make these muscles very susceptible to injury and can also greatly impair your mobility.

If you have poor circulation in your legs due to conditions such as atherosclerosis or diabetes, you will be even more susceptible to developing trigger points in the legs and feet. The more severe the circulation impairment, the more trigger points and pain there will be, and the more severely the ability to exercise will be curtailed, leading to a worsening of the underlying disease.

Some of the more common conditions affecting the calves are muscle strains, compartment syndromes, periosteal irritation (formerly shin splints), cramping, tendinopathies and tendon ruptures, and stress fractures. These can all be caused by trigger points that go undiagnosed and untreated.

Calf Muscle Strains

A *strain* is damage to the muscle fibers, while a *sprain* refers to ligament damage. Strains are "graded" according to the amount of damage. A grade 1 strain is a minor tear, with up to 10 percent of the muscle fibers damaged. Symptoms may include a small amount of pain with tightness and aching for two to five days after the injury, and you can still tolerate using the muscles. A grade 2 strain is damage of up to 90 percent of the muscle fibers, and you will likely feel sharp pain that is worse with walking, along with tightness and aching of the affected area for a week or more, and there will be bruising and swelling. A grade 3 is a full rupture, with more than 90 percent torn muscle fibers. Pain will be severe and there will be a lot of bruising and swelling, and the muscle will bunch up near the top of the calf, which is often described as "a window blind rolling up suddenly."

Calf strains are usually caused by sudden forces being applied to tight calf muscles. You should consider a grade 1 or 2 injury as a warning sign to use the techniques found in this book before you suffer from a complete rupture and possibly require immediate surgery.

Compartment Syndromes

A *muscle compartment* is a group of muscles within a particular part of the body, wrapped by strong, fibrous tissue (*fascia*). The fascia attaches the compartment to the bone, and each compartment has a blood and nerve supply. For example, the lower leg contains four muscle compartments: The superficial posterior (back) compartment contains the soleus and gastrocnemius muscles, and the deep posterior compartment contains the flexor digitorum longus, flexor hallucis longus, popliteus, and posterior tibialis muscles. The anterior (front) compartment contains the tibialis anterior, extensor hallucis longus, extensor digitorum longus, and peroneus tertius. The lateral (outside) compartment contains the peroneus longus and peroneus brevis (see part III for chapters on these muscles, and to see their locations).

A *compartment syndrome* is where increased pressure within the muscle compartment adversely affects blood and lymph circulation of the muscles inside. The most noticeable symptom is tightness, dull aching, and diffuse tenderness over the entire *belly* (the fleshy central part) of the involved muscles. One or more of the muscles swell, causing pain and odd sensations, and the symptoms are worse with activity. Symptoms develop over time, and pain persists for increasing amounts of time after exercise. *It is important to see a doctor immediately.* If left untreated, compartment syndrome eventually causes scarring of the muscles and nerves, and other permanent damage. A positive diagnosis is determined by measuring intramuscular pressure within the compartment. Once it is successfully treated by relieving pressure within the compartment, you should check for trigger points, since they were likely formed as a result of compartment syndrome.

Shin Splints and Tibial Periosteal Stress Syndromes

Anterior compartment syndrome is sometimes called "anterior shin splints," which is easily confused with the generic term "shin splints" used in the past to refer to any chronic pain in the front or middle of the lower leg associated with exercise. More recently, "shin splints" has come to refer specifically to irritation of the surface of the bone along the attachment of a muscle, and is called *periosteal irritation*. In the front of the leg, periosteal irritation may develop when a runner first changes from a flat-footed to a toe-running style, begins training on a track or hill (especially downhill), or runs in a shoe that is either too rigid or too flexible. Trigger point self-help techniques will help resolve periosteal irritation.

Calf Cramps

Calf cramps occur most often when you are sleeping, or sitting for too long with your toes pointed. They are one of the most common symptoms of gastrocnemius trigger points, though other calf muscles may be involved. Calf cramps may also be brought on by dehydration, loss of or inadequate intake of electrolytes (including potassium, calcium, magnesium, and salt), hypoparathyroidism, Parkinson's disease, and possibly diabetes.

If you are experiencing calf cramps, in addition to using the self-help techniques in part III, try increasing your water intake and take a multimineral supplement. If you limit your salt intake severely or sweat heavily, try increasing your salt intake, unless otherwise directed by a doctor. Some drugs can cause calf cramps, such as lithium, cimetidine, bumetanide, vincristine, and phenothiazines. Taking vitamin E (400 IU per day) helps some people a great deal. If you take a multivitamin, be sure to count that amount of vitamin E toward the 400 IU, and take the larger dose for a maximum of two weeks, or less if the cramps disappear more quickly. Try vitamin B$_2$ (riboflavin) if you have calf cramps during pregnancy.

Achilles Tendinopathy and Ruptures

The Achilles is the large tendon at the back of the ankle area that attaches the gastrocnemius and soleus muscles to the heel bone. This tendon enables you to flex and extend your foot, allowing you to walk or run.

As with the other tendinopathies mentioned above, Achilles tendinopathy is caused by micro-trauma to the tendon rather than an inflammatory process. Damage can occur over the course of a few days or over a longer period, depending on your activities.

Symptoms of *acute* Achilles tendinopathy may include pain at the beginning of an exercise that decreases as you continue to exercise, tenderness with pressure applied over the Achilles tendon, and pain that decreases with rest. Symptoms of *chronic* tendinopathy may include pain that develops over a period of weeks or months, pain throughout exercise, pain that is worse when walking uphill or up stairs, pain accompanied by stiffness (particularly in the morning or after resting), tenderness with pressure applied over the tendon, nodules or lumps on the tendon, swelling or thickening over the tendon, and possibly redness on the skin. There is also a bursa on the back of the heel that can become irritated as part of Achilles tendinopathy, a condition called *retrocalcaneal bursitis*. Symptoms may include pain on the back of the heel (especially when running uphill or on soft surfaces), tenderness and swelling, and a spongy resistance when pressing on the area.

Causes of Achilles tendinopathy may include an increase in activity (distance, speed, or hills), change of your footwear or training surface, lack of adequate recovery time between activities, wearing heels (even low ones), foot pronation, weak calf muscles, and tight calf muscles that decrease range of motion at the ankle joint and stress the Achilles tendon. The self-help techniques found in parts II and III of this book will take the stress off the Achilles tendon and allow it to heal.

If the calf muscles are chronically tight and you make abrupt movements, as with sports, you may get a partial or complete Achilles tendon rupture. Symptoms of a partial rupture may include a sudden, sharp pain in the Achilles tendon (or within twenty-four hours of the injury), sharp pains that come back at the beginning of exercise and then again after exercise has stopped, stiffness in the Achilles first thing in the morning, and slight swelling. A total rupture feels as if someone has hit you hard on the calves with something, often accompanied by a loud sound. There will be a large amount of swelling, and you won't be able to walk well or stand on tiptoes. You may need to have surgery within two days in order for the injury to heal properly. Surgery has a lower rerupture rate than nonsurgical options, but all surgeries have risks of complications.

As you have no doubt surmised, it is advisable to treat the calf muscles with self-help techniques before you rupture the tendon. If you have already ruptured the tendon, seek medical treatment and then perform the self-help techniques in this book to prevent reinjury.

Stress Fractures of the Tibia or Fibula

Symptoms of a stress fracture of the tibia (the larger of the two lower-leg bones) may include pain that occurs after running long distances, tenderness and swelling over the site of the fracture (usually in the lower third of the lower leg), and pain when you press on the "shin bone." Stress fractures of the fibula (the smaller of the two bones) are less common, and the pain will be located more over the outside of the lower leg rather than over the tibia.

Causes of tibial fractures include overloading the bones by long-distance running, a sudden change in running surface, and numerous cumulative small impacts to the bones. Causes of fibular fractures include tightness of the muscles surrounding the bone placing torque on the bone, and foot pronation. Using the techniques found in this book will help prevent fractures, and will also help heal and prevent further injury if you have had a fracture.

Deep Vein Thrombosis

Deep vein thrombosis (DVT) is a blood clot in a vein, most commonly in the calf, which is most likely to occur after surgery or a long airplane ride. You are more at risk for DVT if you are over fifty, have poor circulation, or are overweight. It is potentially fatal if the clot works its way loose and travels to the heart, lung, or brain. Symptoms may include constant calf pain, swelling, heat in the area, deep tenderness in the muscle, and sometimes a localized reddening of the skin. If you think you are experiencing the symptoms of DVT, you should not receive massage of any kind, and you should seek medical help immediately for evaluation. Do NOT perform the techniques on the calf muscles found in this book, as pressure can help loosen the clot.

Ankle and Foot Pain

Your ankles and feet support the weight of your entire body. They are your foundation, shock absorbers, balance mechanism, and means of getting around. One-quarter of the bones in the human body (twenty-six) are in the feet. There are thirty-three joints, and more than one hundred muscles, tendons, and ligaments. A problem that develops in the ankles and feet affects the entire body, for example when you limp or have to be on crutches while healing.

The most common problems affecting the ankles and feet are sprains, muscle and tendon tightness and subsequent damage, tibialis posterior syndrome, plantar fasciitis, stress fractures, hallux valgus, and toe drop.

Ankle Sprains

It is estimated that between twenty-three and twenty-seven thousand lateral ankle sprains occur daily in the United States alone, though actual occurrences are probably significantly higher because as many as 55 percent of people with sprains may not seek treatment from a health care professional. Once an ankle has been sprained, the chance of spraining it again is greater than 70 percent, due to the injury to multiple structures in the ankle as well as changes in the central nervous system function that maintains a balance-feedback system, known as the "sensimotor system" (Wickstrom and Cordova 2009).

The most common ankle sprain is due to stretching or tearing of the lateral (outer side) ligaments. It is possible to sprain the medial ligament (located on the "medial" side of the ankle, which is the side facing the other ankle), but that occurs more often in conjunction with a fracture. Sprained ankles, as with all ligament sprains, are divided into grades 1, 2, or 3, depending on their severity.

Mild sprains may cause only some discomfort. The more severe the sprain, the more swelling and bruising, pain, and joint instability. If your ankle is severely sprained, you may have ruptured ligaments and dislocated the ankle joint. There may also be damage to the tendons and other joint tissues, and small fractures, so you may need to get an X-ray to determine the extent of damage.

Foot pronation and supination may make you more susceptible to ankle sprains, so flat shoes with wide bases (no heels) are advisable, along with orthotics that stabilize your foot (see part II).

Calf muscles tighten up in response to an ankle sprain, so you will want to do the self-help techniques contained in part III of this book to relieve tightness and prevent future injuries.

Peroneal Muscle and Tendon Damage

The peroneus longus, brevis and tertius are found along the outside of the lower leg. Symptoms of tendinopathy here may include swelling on the outside of the ankle or heel, and pain that increases with activity, when pressure is applied over the tendons, and when your foot is moved in certain directions. Causes include running on side-slanted surfaces (such as a road), overuse, foot pronation, and tight calf muscles, particularly the peroneal muscles. An ankle sprain can cause the peroneal tendons to slip forward over the outer ankle bone (lateral malleolus). A tight peroneus brevis muscle can cause a rupture of the tendon. Focus on the peroneal muscle chapter in part III and see the section "Self-help technique: Choose appropriate footwear" in chapter 4. Self-help techniques will help prevent injuries.

Tibialis Posterior Syndrome

Tibialis posterior syndrome is another tendinopathy. The tibialis posterior is on the back of the leg, "deep to" the gastrocnemius and soleus; that is, it's the muscle right next to the tibia and fibula bones. Pain will most likely be felt on the bottom of the foot, and there may be swelling around the middle ankle bone (medial malleolus). Foot pronation predisposes you to this injury, which is easily corrected with good orthotics and shoes with good heel bases. Do the self-help techniques found in part III to relax the tibialis posterior muscle belly, which will help relax the tendon.

Plantar Fasciitis, Heel Pain, and Heel Spurs

Heel pain can be caused by a number of conditions, including a bruised or even fractured heel (caused by repetitive pounding as in running), calcaneal bursitis, tarsal tunnel syndrome, plantar fasciitis, or referred pain from calf muscles, primarily the soleus. By far the most common sources of heel pain are plantar fasciitis and trigger points, and their relationship to each other. Unfortunately, many practitioners aren't familiar with trigger points, so the true source of heel pain goes undiagnosed and untreated.

Plantar Fasciitis

Contrary to its name ("-itis") and what was originally thought, plantar fasciitis is not an inflammatory process, but rather is caused by tension overload on the *plantar aponeurosis* (the flat, broad tendons found between your heel and the ball of your foot) fascial attachment on the big bone in the heel. This tension overload is caused by tightness in the gastrocnemius, soleus, abductor hallucis, flexor digitorum brevis, and/or abductor digiti minimi muscles. The quadratus plantae may also be involved.

Pain from plantar fasciitis develops gradually but will initially be more noticeable after an increase in athletic activity. Pain is worse in the morning, with your first steps being extremely painful until the muscles and plantar fascia have been stretched. Pain often is worse again in the evening, and after running or jumping. Foot pronation adds to the problem.

Treating trigger points, receiving ultrasound, and getting good orthotics with arch supports and deep heel cups are effective therapies. You will need to avoid running, jumping, and possibly walking until symptoms have decreased. You may need to lose weight, since additional weight puts a lot of stress on the lower leg and foot structures. Numerous repeated injections of steroids can lead to rupture of the plantar aponeurosis, so you should use the above treatments first. The longer the condition goes on and the more you limp, the more muscles get involved, all the way up through the back and neck, so you should not wait to start treatment.

Heel Spurs

A heel spur is a little extra piece of bone that forms somewhere on the *calcaneus*, or heel bone, on the side closer to the arches of your foot. You may have heel spurs with no pain, and plantar fasciitis and heel pain with no heel spurs, but they often come together. Plantar fasciitis was thought for a number of years to cause heel spur formation, but a 2007 study (Li and Muehleman) presented a compelling argument against heel spur formation being caused by traction from the plantar aponeurosis and muscle attachments. By studying cadavers with heel spurs, including examining the direction of the spur bone fibers (*trabeculae*), the location of the spurs, and the variability of muscle and fiber attachments (or lack thereof) to the spur, the researchers determined it was unlikely that heel spurs were formed by traction from these tissues pulling on the heel. Based on their findings, they hypothesized that heel spurs more likely formed as a result of *vertical loading*, or pressure from above, and spurs actually serve the function of protecting the heel bone from developing microfractures. They also noted a pattern of an increasing number of heel spurs with age, and that for most people, heel stress would be a result of excessive force over a period of years, in addition to the individual variability in the arches and other foot structures. They also noted that, for non-athletes, increased *body mass index* (a measure of body fat based on the ratio of height and weight) plus a spur were two main factors in heel pain. If their hypothesis is correct, spurs would form in response to an increasing body mass, so gaining weight alone could account for both the heel pain and the spur formation independently.

Stress Fractures

Several bones in the foot are susceptible to stress fractures, including the navicular, calcaneus (heel), and metatarsal bones. Symptoms may include pain that is worse during an activity, and possibly swelling and tenderness at the site of the fracture. You can probably still walk, and an X-ray might not necessarily be diagnostic, since stress fractures might not be visible on an X-ray. A bone scan or MRI might be necessary. Stress fractures are caused by prolonged, repeated loads such as running, hiking long distances, or being overweight. Tight calf and foot muscles are also likely involved, so the self-help techniques in this book will be helpful for preventing future injuries.

Foot Tendinopathies

There are numerous tendons in your foot that attach at various places, allowing you to flex and extend both your foot and toes. The most common symptom of foot tendinopathies is pain, though there may also be some swelling. A variety of problems can cause foot tendinopathies, including improper footwear, overuse, foot pronation, being overweight, and tight muscles in the calf and foot. The best way to resolve this problem is to wear proper shoes (addressed further in part II), apply the self-help techniques found in this book to relieve muscle tightness, and, if necessary, lose weight.

Claw Toes, Hammertoes, and Mallet Toe

These conditions are associated with long-standing tightness of the toe's long extensor muscles, and often tight calf muscles too. With all three conditions, your toes are bent up at one of the toe's joints. A person with claw toe (or claw foot) also has high arches, giving the foot a clawlike appearance. Self-help techniques may give at least partial relief, and proper footwear is essential to prevent further aggravation and deformity.

Bunions and Hallux Valgus

Hallux valgus is a painful condition where the big toe becomes displaced and deformed. Tightness and trigger points in the flexor hallucis longus muscle can help cause hallux valgus, and the more the bone has spread, the more force is exerted by the muscle on the bone, making the cycle self-perpetuating. The flexor hallucis brevis, adductor hallucis and abductor hallucis (the superficial intrinsic foot muscles covered in chapter 23) become weak, allowing even further spread. A *bunion*, or swelling of the protective lubricating pad on the side of the big toe, can form and cause additional pain.

It is important to avoid high heels during childhood and teenage bone-formative years to drastically reduce the likelihood of developing bunions later in life. Relief of trigger points may stop the progression or even reverse some of the spread of hallux valgus and subsequent bunions, though surgery may be necessary if the condition has progressed far enough. Proper footwear and orthotics are essential if you have either of these conditions.

Toe Drop

Toe drop is caused by trigger points in the tibialis anterior muscle. You aren't able to lift your foot up when walking (plantar flexion), so you may trip or fall. Trigger points in the tibialis anterior can be caused by acute injuries or walking up or down hills when you aren't used to nonlevel surfaces. See part III for treatment of this condition.

Conclusion

In this chapter, you have learned about the many causes of leg and foot pain, and their relationship to trigger points—both how tight muscles can make you susceptible to injuries and chronic problems, and how injuries and chronic problems can lead to the formation of trigger points and lead to a self-perpetuating cycle of pain.

The next part of the book lists common factors than can cause trigger points and keep them activated. It will help you figure out why you have developed trigger points and offer additional suggestions for dealing with these perpetuating factors.

Part II

WHAT CAUSES TRIGGER POINTS AND KEEPS THEM GOING: PERPETUATING FACTORS

If we treat myofascial pain syndromes without…correcting the multiple perpetuating factors, the patient is doomed to endless cycles of treatment and relapse… Usually, one stress activates the [trigger point], then other factors perpetuate it. In some patients, these perpetuating factors are so important that their elimination results in complete relief of the pain without any local treatment.

—Doctors Janet Travell and David G. Simons (1983, 103)

This section outlines some general causes that activate or perpetuate trigger points and offers many suggestions on how to address the perpetuating factors to help you eliminate lower leg, knee, ankle, or foot pain. (In part III, the chapters on individual muscles will give you additional suggestions specific to each muscle.) I recommend you read each chapter to learn how body mechanics, diet, and other perpetuating factors may contribute to your pain. Multiple factors are often involved, and up to this point, you may not have been aware that these factors could be contributing to your pain. Common perpetuating factors include mechanical stressors, injuries, spinal misalignments, nutrient deficiencies, poor dietary habits, food allergies, emotional factors, sleep problems, acute or chronic infections, hormonal imbalances, and organ dysfunction and disease.

As you address perpetuating factors, pace yourself so that the process isn't too overwhelming. Work on your perpetuating factors over time. You probably can't make all the needed changes at once. As you begin to address your perpetuating factors, go ahead and start on the self-help techniques in part III. Applying pressure to trigger points will probably relieve pain and other symptoms either temporarily or for the long term; however, it won't resolve the underlying perpetuating factors. If you get temporary relief from trigger point therapy but your symptoms quickly recur, then trigger points are definitely a factor, but you'll need to address perpetuating factors to gain more lasting relief.

Chapter 4

Body Mechanics

How you sit, stand, walk, run, move, and generally treat your muscles has a great influence on whether or not you form or perpetuate trigger points. Properly fitting shoes, furniture that fits and supports you, and modification of certain activities will greatly speed your healing and help provide long-term relief. Even learning proper posture, especially head positioning, is critical to treating trigger points, since head-forward posture can cause and perpetuate trigger points all the way down into the legs and feet. Treating new injuries promptly can help prevent the formation of trigger points, and the treatment of older injuries, as well as spinal misalignments and other problems in the skeletal system, can help stop the perpetuation of trigger points.

Mechanical Stressors

Chronic mechanical stressors such as wearing improperly fitting or worn-out shoes, playing sports without proper warm-up, standing or sitting for long periods, and skeletal asymmetries cause a self-perpetuating cycle of trigger point aggravation. They are among the most common causes and perpetuators of trigger points involved in lower leg, knee, ankle, or foot pain. Fortunately most are nearly always correctable, and minimizing or eliminating them is one of the most important things you can do to break your cycle of pain.

Abuse of Muscles

Playing sports can cause trigger points due to a number of factors: improper warm-up, overusing certain muscles or muscle groups while underusing others, receiving direct blows to body parts, strains and sprains, tendon ruptures, and fractures. You are particularly susceptible if you are a "weekend warrior" and do strenuous athletic activities only a day or two per week.

Your posture can also affect your entire body. If you slouch at your desk or on your couch, or if you read in bed, your muscles will suffer, all the way down into your legs and feet. Abuse of muscles includes poor body mechanics (such as lifting improperly), long periods of immobility (such as sitting at a desk or standing without a break), repetitive movements (such as scooting your chair around using your legs), and holding your body in awkward positions for long periods, such as squatting. The self-help techniques listed below will help you prevent abuse of your muscles.

Self-help technique: Train and warm up properly for sports. Stretch adequately before each activity, cross-train so you build up all muscles, and increase distance, repetitions, and weights gradually to reduce risk of injury.

Self-help technique: Be aware of your body mechanics. Be sure to sit while putting clothing on your lower body. This can go a long way toward preventing additional injuries in your legs and feet, and also helps you avoid falls. Also, learn to lift properly using your knees, not your back.

Self-help technique: Take frequent breaks. Anytime you must sit, stand, or squat for long periods, take frequent breaks. One good trick is to set a timer across the room; you'll have to get up to turn it off.

Misfitting Furniture

Misfitting furniture is a major cause of muscular pain, particularly in the workplace. Sitting at a desk or computer, whether at work or home, places a great deal of stress on your muscles, which can affect your body all the way down to your feet. Sitting in a chair that places uneven pressure on the back of your thighs causes trigger points in your hamstring muscles, and a chair that doesn't allow you to put your feet level on the ground causes trigger points in your lower leg and foot muscles. But there are many things you can do to improve your office setup, and many of them aren't too expensive, such as lumbar supports, phone headsets, and copyholders. Just sticking a thick catalog under your computer screen to raise it to the proper height can make a big difference. Having these gadgets readily available will ensure you use them as much as possible.

Get Office Furniture That Fits You

Modifying or replacing misfitting furniture is one of the easiest things you can do to help get relief from trigger points. Once it's done, you won't have to do it on a daily or frequent basis as part of your self-help. You'll still need to be aware of your posture, but furniture that corrects some of your counterproductive postural habits without you having to be aware of them is much simpler. Consider contacting a company that specializes in ergonomics to come to your workplace and assess your office arrangement. They can make some adjustments and help you select furniture that fits your body. Your employer may balk at the cost, but if you end up with health problems as a result of a poor workstation, they'll end up paying for it in lost work time and workers' compensation claims. If your employer won't pay for this, consider paying for it yourself. What is it worth to you to be pain free?

Chair. Your elbows and forearms should rest evenly on either your work surface or armrests of the proper height. The armrests must be high enough to support your elbows without you leaning to the side, but not so high as to cause your shoulders to hike up. The upholstery needs to be firm, and casters should be avoided, since scooting your chair around causes and perpetuates leg and foot trigger points. Your knees should fit under your desk, and your chair needs to be close enough that you can lean against your backrest. A good chair supports both your lumbar area and your midback, and has a backrest with a slope slightly back from vertical. The seat should be low enough that your feet rest flat on the floor without compression of your thighs by the front edge of the seat, high enough that not all the pressure is placed on your gluteal area, and slightly hollowed out to accommodate your buttocks. If you cannot sit at the proper height for your desk and computer as well as rest your feet on the floor, you may need to get a footstool in order to avoid compression of your hamstring muscles. If you look around, you can get a good adjustable chair for around $120.

Computer screen. Your computer screen should be directly in front of you, slightly below eye level and slightly tilted back at the top. If you work from hard copy, attach it to the side of the screen with a copyholder so that you can look directly forward as much as possible rather than tipping your head down or turning it too far to the side. You can raise the height of your screen by placing catalogs or books underneath it until it's at the correct level. Evaluate your workstation to make sure that you don't have glare on your screen, that your lighting is adequate, and that your computer screen isn't bothering your eyes.

Keyboard and mouse. Your keyboard and mouse should be kept as close to lap level as possible. An ergonomically correct keyboard and keyboard tray allow you to keep the keyboard near your lap and use your chair armrests while typing. I see a lot of what I call "mouse injuries," that is, arm and shoulder pain due to using a computer mouse for extended periods without proper arm support.

Headset. A telephone headset can provide a great deal of relief from neck and back pain, which can affect you all the way into your feet. Telephone shoulder rests aren't adequate, and if you try to hold the phone in your hand, you'll end up cradling it between your head and shoulder at some point, which is very hard on your neck and trapezius muscles. Get headsets for all of your phones—at work, at home, and for your cell phone.

Lumbar support. A lumbar support helps correct round-shouldered posture. Most chiropractic offices carry lumbar supports of varying thickness. I recommend that you get one for your car and one for your favorite seat at home. Try to avoid sitting on anything without back support, since this causes you to sit with your shoulders and upper back slumped forward. When going to sporting events, picnics, or other places where you won't have back support, bring a Crazy Creek–brand chair or something similar to provide at least some support. You can get one through most major sporting goods suppliers. They cost only about forty dollars—a good investment in your back— and they're very lightweight for carrying. Or consider a lightweight collapsible chair, also available at sporting goods stores.

Bedtime Furniture

You probably spend about one-third of your time in bed, so it is extremely important to make sure your pillows and bed are right for you. Sleeping on a couch or in a chair should definitely be avoided.

Pillows. If your pillow is made from foam rubber or some other springy material that will jiggle your neck, get rid of it! Vibrations from these pillows will aggravate trigger points in the back and neck. (However, memory foam pillows are fine.) Your pillow should support your head at a level that keeps your spine in alignment and is comfortable when you are lying on your side. Chiropractic offices usually carry well-designed pillows. I always take my pillow with me when I travel; that way I know I have something comfortable to sleep on, and it comes in handy if I get stuck in an airport.

Bed. A bed that is too soft can cause a lot of muscular problems. You may not even realize that your bed is too soft. People usually insist their mattress is firm enough, but when queried further they admit that sleeping on a mat on the floor gives them relief when their pain is particularly bad. Try putting a camping mat on the floor and sleeping on it for a week. If you feel better, your mattress isn't firm enough, no matter how much money you spent on it or how well it worked for someone else. Different people need different kinds of mattresses. An all-cotton futon is very firm and may be best for some people. Mattresses really last only about five to seven years, and after that time they should be replaced. Also consider that if your partner is heavier, you may be unaware that you brace yourself slightly in order not to roll into him or her. Some types of mattresses can accommodate couples who need different degrees of firmness.

Clothing

You may be surprised to learn that what you wear and how you wear it can cause or perpetuate trigger points. Since constricting clothing can impair circulation, it can directly cause trigger points. Footwear is the most important clothing item to pay attention to if you have pain anywhere in your legs and feet. Anytime you're standing or walking, your feet affect your entire posture and gait. High heels and other footwear with heels can cause muscular tension throughout your body, thereby contributing to trigger points. Fortunately clothing is a problem that's easily correctable, as you see in the self-help techniques below.

Self-help technique: Choose appropriate footwear and get orthotics. Don't wear high heels, cowboy boots, or other shoes with heels.

While correcting foot supination (more weight on the inside of your foot) or pronation (more weight on the outside of your foot) is essential for some people, almost everyone can benefit from using some kind of foot support inserted in their shoes. Shoes rarely have adequate arch support, and this affects muscles all the way up through your body. My favorite noncorrective orthotics are the Superfeet brand. They have a deep heel cup, which helps prevent pronation and supination, and they provide excellent arch support. Superfeet has a variety of models, including cheaper, noncustom trim-to-fit insoles and moderately priced custom-molded insoles. Their products can provide support in a wide variety of footwear. Visit superfeet.com to learn more about their products. If you find you need corrective orthotics, you will need to see a podiatrist.

Self-help technique: Loosen your clothing. Constricting clothing can lead to impaired circulation and muscular problems. My rule of thumb is if clothing leaves an elastic mark or indentation on your skin, it is too tight and is cutting off proper circulation. Check your socks, belts, waistbands, bras, and ties to see if they're too tight. Tight waistbands and socks in particular can cause and perpetuate trigger points in the legs and feet.

Self-help technique: Carry your purse or daypack properly. If you carry a purse, get one with a long strap and put the strap over your head so you wear it diagonally across your torso rather than over one shoulder, and keep its contents light. If you use a daypack, put the straps over both shoulders. When you carry a purse or pack over one shoulder, you have to hike up that shoulder at least a little to keep the strap from slipping off, no matter how light your purse or pack may be. When you are leaning to one side on top, you are putting unequal stress on your legs and feet.

Head-Forward Posture

Head-forward posture leads to the development and perpetuation of trigger points throughout the entire body. If you doubt this, take your shoes off and stand in the position in the second photo below, with your head over your shoulders. Notice how your legs and feet feel—both the pressure distribution and which muscles you are using. Now jut your head forward just a little bit and notice what happens in your legs and feet. If you are not sure whether you chronically hold your head forward, stand in a position that is normal for you, and have someone look at your side profile to see if your head is farther forward than your trunk. The farther you hold your head forward of your shoulders, the more trigger points you're likely to develop (Marcus et al. 1999). Postural exercises can help eliminate head-forward posture.

Self-help technique: Use lumbar support. Poor posture while sitting—whether in a car, at a desk, in front of a computer, or while eating dinner or watching TV—can cause or aggravate head-forward posture. Using a good lumbar support everywhere you sit will help correct poor sitting posture and, ultimately, head-forward posture.

Self-help technique: Do postural exercises. To develop proper posture and reduce head-forward posture, stand with your feet about four inches apart, with your arms at your sides and your thumbs pointing forward. Tighten your buttocks to stabilize your lower back, and then, while inhaling, rotate your arms and shoulders out and back (rotating your thumbs backward) and squeeze your shoulder blades closer together behind you. While holding this position, drop your shoulders down and exhale. Move your head back to bring your ears in line with your shoulders, and hold this position for about six seconds while breathing normally. (When moving your head, don't tilt your head up or down or open your mouth.) Relax, but try to maintain good posture once you release the pose. If holding this position feels uncomfortable or stiff, try shifting your weight from your heels to the balls of your feet, which will cause your head to move backward over your shoulders. Repeat this exercise frequently throughout the day to develop good posture. Do it every hour or two. It is better to do one repetition six or more times per day than to do six repetitions in a row (Travell and Simons 1983).

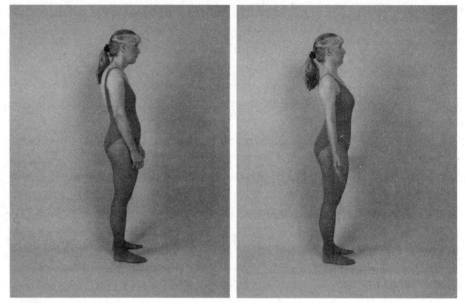

Skeletal Asymmetries

A skeletal asymmetry, including a shorter leg and a smaller *hemipelvis* on one side (the left or right portion of the pelvis), can contribute to trigger points in the lower leg, knee, ankle, or foot. Fortunately these can be corrected inexpensively and noninvasively with a pad that goes in one shoe or a pad that goes on your chair under one buttock. (In this book, the term "shorter leg" refers to an anatomical leg length inequality, where the bones are actually shorter on one side, rather than the "shorter leg" caused by a spinal misalignment, which is a term chiropractors use when one hip is higher than the other, giving the appearance of one leg being shorter than the other.) Other skeletal disproportions can also be corrected. For example, a long second toe can be corrected with shoe orthotics, and short upper arms can be corrected with ergonomically correct furniture.

Injuries

Injuries are one of the most common initiators of trigger points in general, and in lower leg, knee, ankle, and foot muscles specifically. A healthy muscle is pliable to the touch when not in use but will feel firm if called upon for action. If a muscle feels firm at rest, it is tight in an unhealthy way, even if you work out.

I like to use an analogy of a rubber band and a stick. If a sudden, unexpected force is applied to a stick, it's likely to be damaged, and the same is true of a tight muscle, where the force could be something like a fall or a car accident. If, however, a sudden force is applied to a rubber band, it will stretch to absorb the force instead, and the same is true of a pliable, healthy muscle, making it much less likely to be injured. A muscle may be tight and restricted without you being aware of it, since latent trigger points restrict range of motion to some degree and almost everyone has some latent trigger points. These muscles containing latent trigger points can be injured easily if a sudden force is applied.

New Injuries

Treating an injury when it first occurs can prevent trigger points from forming and help you avoid an escalating cycle of pain. See an acupuncturist or massage therapist who is experienced in working with recent injuries. You may also need to see a chiropractor or osteopathic physician.

Surgeries and Scars

A surgery is likely to leave some scar tissue, which can perpetuate trigger points. Scar tissue can be broken up, to an extent, with vigorous cross-friction massage, a technique in which you rub both of your thumbs in opposing directions back and forth across the scar. However, most people won't work on their own scars vigorously enough due to the pain it causes. You will probably need to see a practitioner for help. Acupuncture can treat scar tissue and help eliminate the pain from trigger points around the area. I recommend using both cross-friction massage and acupuncture rather than just one or the other.

Self-Help Techniques for Acute Injuries and Post-Surgery Recovery

RICE:

- **Rest** the affected body part.

- **Ice** can reduce swelling, help prevent bruising, and increase blood flow to the area. You can use a cold compress (cold water with ice cubes in a gallon baggie works well). Or, if it is your lower leg or foot, you can submerge it in ice water to your tolerance for a length of time; you can put your foot or leg in and take it out as needed. Ice off and on for at least 48 hours.

- **Compression,** such as with an ace bandage (but not so tight as to cut off circulation!). This technique is for acute injuries only, unless otherwise instructed by your medical provider.

- **Elevation** of the affected area reduces bleeding and swelling.

Also:

- Gentle massage strokes on the skin, stroking toward your heart, will improve circulation.

- Cross-friction massage and acupuncture are helpful in healing and reducing scar tissue after swelling and bruising have disappeared.

Buy:

- Get some arnica or Traumeel ointment and oral homeopathics from your local health food stores.

- There are Chinese herbs for traumatic injury, which you can get from your local acupuncture practitioner. Naturopathic doctors will also have herbs and trauma kits.

Have these handy in your medicine cabinet in case of unexpected acute injuries, and also if you are planning to have a surgery. They work best when use is started immediately after the injury, and as soon after surgery as possible.

Skeletal Misalignments and Spinal Problems

If vertebrae in your back are chronically out of alignment, the stress placed on muscles due to tightness and pain can cause trigger points to form, which will affect your body all the way down to your toes. Be aware that you may also suffer from misalignments in your hip joints and leg, ankle, and foot bones. These are usually caused by tight muscles to begin with, so a combined approach of skeletal adjustments plus massage or acupuncture is probably necessary for lasting relief.

Skeletal adjustments can be performed by a chiropractor or osteopathic physician, but be sure you choose one who adjusts bones in extremities, since some do only spinal adjustments. They will likely take X-rays at the initial visit to evaluate your spine. If you have already had X-rays taken, bring them with you so you can avoid the additional cost and exposure to radiation involved in duplicating X-rays.

Chronic pain from herniated and bulging disks may also lead to formation of trigger points in your entire body, because it probably affects the way you move and walk. Herniated and bulging disks can be very successfully treated with acupuncture (especially plum blossom technique), but if you don't get some relief fairly quickly, you may want to consider surgery. Spinal surgery has gotten so sophisticated that many surgeries are fairly minor procedures that have you back on your feet the next day. If you have *stenosis* (a narrowing of the central spinal cord canal or the holes where the nerves come out), acupuncture will help with pain but not the stenosis, so surgery may be the best option. With any surgery there is a certain amount of risk, so be sure to discuss this with your operating physician and make sure you understand the procedure. If you are still unsure, get a second opinion from another surgeon. Disk problems and stenosis must be confirmed with an MRI. If you have surgery but your pain continues, trigger points are likely to be the culprit, in which case they need to be treated so you can experience lasting relief. If you still don't get relief, the pain may be due to scar tissue from the surgery compressing a nerve root, something you'll need to confirm with your doctor.

Bone spurs and narrowed disk spaces can also cause chronic pain and lead to the formation of trigger points. But in a random sample of the population, you will find many people with bone spurs and narrowed disk spaces who don't experience pain, and many people who do experience pain but don't have bone spurs or narrowed disk spaces. Don't assume these are causing your problems, even if a practitioner has made this assumption.

I always start with the premise that trigger points are at least part of the problem, if not all of the problem, and treat accordingly. If a patient doesn't get some relief fairly quickly, then I know something else may be going on. At that point, I refer them to someone who can evaluate them with an X-ray or MRI.

Conclusion

To address perpetuating factors related to body mechanics, start with changing your footwear and getting noncustom orthotics. Notice how you are using your body, particularly during sports, and be sure not to overdo new exercises. Stretch well before and after athletic activities. Notice how you hold your body, and start retraining yourself to both relax and learn proper posture. Something that may initially seem irrelevant to your situation may lead to a dramatic reduction in the intensity and frequency of your pain. If the self-help techniques aren't effective, consult with a health care professional who can help you figure out which self-help approaches are most important for you, or to get fitted for custom corrective devices.

The next chapter will discuss nutrition and other dietary perpetuating factors. Obesity, which affects your body both mechanically and systemically, will be discussed in chapter 6.

Chapter 5

Diet

What you eat and drink has a great deal to do with the perpetuation of trigger points. Improving your nutrition, drinking enough water, and avoiding certain foods, drinks, and other substances can greatly decrease trigger point aggravation, and therefore also decrease both the intensity and frequency of your lower leg, knee, ankle, or foot pain.

Nutritional Deficiencies

It is easy and relatively inexpensive to improve your nutrient intake to see if it will decrease your symptoms. Doctors Travell and Simons (1983) found that almost half of their patients required treatment for vitamin deficiencies to obtain lasting relief from the pain and dysfunction of trigger points. They believed it was one of the most important perpetuating factors to address. The more deficient in nutrients you are, the more symptoms of all kinds. Even if a blood test shows that you're at the low end of the normal range for a given vitamin or mineral, it's possible that you need more of it, since your body pulls certain nutrients from your tissues before it allows a decrease in blood levels of those nutrients.

Several factors may lead to nutrient insufficiency, including inadequate intake of a nutrient, impaired nutrient absorption, inadequate nutrient utilization, increased need by the body, nutrients leaving the body too quickly, and nutrients being destroyed within the body too quickly.

What to Take

Even if you have a fairly healthy diet, you may need supplements. In many places, agricultural soils have been depleted of nutrients by repeatedly planting the same crops in the same location rather than rotating them to replenish the soil. Use of chemical fertilizers and pesticides can also adversely affect both crops and soil, so food doesn't always provide all of the nutrition we require. Shipping food over long distances or storing it for long periods also depletes the nutritive value—too much time passes between when the crop is picked and when it is consumed. Most people need to take some kind of multivitamin and multimineral supplement to ensure proper nutrition, especially those who fall into one of the high-risk groups mentioned below.

Don't megadose on supplements unless a doctor has determined your condition warrants it, since taking too much of certain vitamins, such as A, D, E, and folic acid, can actually be detrimental and could cause symptoms similar to deficiencies. You may want to work with a practitioner to develop a personalized supplement program. Some health care providers can arrange for testing to determine any inadequacies. This is especially important because some people aren't able to absorb certain nutrients and need to take them in megadoses or have them injected. For example, some people can't absorb vitamin B_{12}, so they need to get intramuscular injections to ensure adequate levels.

The sections below will discuss the nutrients most likely to be involved in the perpetuation of trigger points. If you have other nutritional concerns or would like more information about any of the nutrients discussed here, *Prescription for Nutritional Healing* by James F. Balch, MD, and Phyllis A. Balch, CNC (2000) is an excellent source. It offers information on vitamins, minerals, amino acids, antioxidants, and enzymes, and it lists food sources for each. Sections on common disorders list supplements useful for treating each condition.

Self-help technique: Take supplements. Because some vitamins require the presence of other vitamins for optimal absorption or effectiveness, taking a good multivitamin supplement and a good multimineral supplement helps ensure that the needed combinations are present. If you take a multivitamin that also includes minerals, be sure to check the label to make sure there are adequate amounts of minerals in it; if not, you may need to take a multimineral too. In addition, you might need to take supplements of some of the vitamins and minerals listed below. Doctors Travell and Simons (1983) found that the most important supplements for treating trigger points were the water-soluble vitamins C, B_1, B_6, B_{12}, and folic acid, and the minerals calcium, magnesium, iron, and potassium.

When to Take Supplements

Take your vitamins with food, since some nutrients need to bind with substances found in food in order to be absorbed. You may find that it is best to take your vitamins and herbs when you are not sick, with the exception of herbs specifically made for fighting illness. Some pathogens can get stronger from some vitamins and herbs, and you could get sicker. (See "Acute or Chronic Infections" in chapter 6 for suggestions on how to head off illness.) Once all of your symptoms have abated, you can resume your regular program of supplementation.

Impaired Digestive Function and Nutrient Malabsorption

If your digestive system isn't functioning well, symptoms may include any of the following: gas, belching, bloating, acid regurgitation, heartburn, diarrhea, constipation, pencil-thin stools, undigested food in your stools, and weight gain even though you're not eating excessively. Taking digestive enzymes or hydrochloric acid for long periods isn't a good solution for poor digestion, because they can take over some of the natural digestive functions of your body. Instead, you need to repair your body so it can do its job properly. A naturopath, acupuncturist, or herbalist can help you figure out whether you have digestive problems. These professionals can also give you dietary recommendations based on your unique constitution as well as any health problems you might have, and can prescribe herbs to rebalance your system.

Although fasting is often recommended as a way to give the digestive system a rest, it's actually hard on the digestive system. If you want to do a cleanse, use herbs and psyllium, but don't stop eating. Another common misconception is that raw foods and whole grains are the healthiest things to eat. For most foods, it's actually better to cook (not overcook!) them to start the chemical breakdown process so your digestive system doesn't have to work as hard. If you have digestive difficulties, white rice and white bread are easier to digest than whole grain products. As your digestive function heals, your practitioner can recommend the appropriate foods for your constitution.

If you have chronic diarrhea, food won't remain in your intestines long enough for nutrients to be adequately absorbed. You will need to identify and eliminate the source of diarrhea. Acupuncture, herbs, and dietary changes can often successfully address this problem.

I've seen many people who have injured their digestive system by taking too many herbs, or herbs that are inappropriate for their health conditions and constitution. Most herbs should be taken only with the advice of a qualified practitioner. An herb that's beneficial for a friend or a family member may not be appropriate for you.

High-Risk Groups

You may be at a higher risk for nutrient deficiency if you are elderly, pregnant or nursing, poor, depressed, or seriously ill, or if you abuse alcohol or other drugs. If you tend to diet by leaving out important food groups or have an eating disorder, you are also likely to have nutrient deficiencies. And in general, many of us have diets that are neither balanced nor high in nutrition. If you eat a lot of processed foods, be aware that they don't contain as much nutrition as foods that are freshly prepared.

Vegetarianism and Nutrition

Most people should not be strict vegetarians. The forms of B_6 found in animal sources are more stable and less likely to be damaged or lost during cooking or preserving than the main form found in plants. In addition, vitamin B_{12} is found only in animal proteins, including dairy products. Even brewer's yeast doesn't contain B_{12} unless the yeast is grown on a special substrate that contains it.

Self-help technique: Improve your protein intake. If you're vegetarian, at the very least you should eat organic eggs, as they are a source of high-quality protein. Most vegetarians are not very good about combining foods to optimize the balance of amino acids (the constituents of protein) in their diet. Even if they are, many report feeling better within a few months when they add high-quality animal protein back into their diet, even if it is just a few eggs or a piece of fish once per week or a couple of times per month.

Vitamins

Adequate intake of vitamin C and the B vitamins is important for resolving trigger points. The B complex vitamins should be taken together, since they rely on each other for proper absorption and use by your body.

Vitamin C

Vitamin C reduces postexercise soreness and strengthens the capillaries; when these tiny blood vessels are fragile, you'll bruise easily. (Hint: If you don't remember how you got a bruise, you're probably bruising too easily.) Vitamin C is essential for the formation of collagen (connective tissue) and bones, and is required for synthesis of the neurotransmitters norepinephrine and serotonin. It is needed for your body's response to stress, plays an important role in immune system function, and decreases the irritability of trigger points caused by infection. Vitamin C helps with diarrhea due to food allergies, but taking too much can lead to watery diarrhea or nonspecific urethritis.

Initial symptoms of vitamin C deficiency include weakness, lethargy, irritability, vague aching pains in the joints and muscles, easy bruising, and possibly weight loss. With severe deficiency (scurvy), the gums become red and swollen and bleed easily, and the teeth may become loose or fall out; however, this condition is rare in most countries with ample access to fruits and vegetables. Vitamin C is likely to be deficient in smokers, alcoholics, older people (the presence of vitamin C in the tissues decreases with age), infants fed primarily on cows' milk (usually between the ages of six and twelve months), people with chronic diarrhea, psychiatric patients, and fad dieters.

Self-help technique: Get enough vitamin C. Good food sources include citrus fruits and fresh juices, raw broccoli, raw brussels sprouts, collard greens, kale, turnip greens, guava, raw sweet peppers, cabbage, and potatoes. It is currently known that vitamin C daily doses above 400 milligrams (mg) are not used by the body, and that taking 1,000 mg daily increases the risk of kidney stones in people with kidney problems, so megadosing with vitamin C is not necessary (Simons, Travell, and Simons 1999, 207). Women taking estrogen or oral contraceptives may need 500 mg per day. Do not take vitamin C together with antacids. Since vitamin C is ascorbic acid and the purpose of an antacid is to neutralize acid, antacids will neutralize vitamin C and make it ineffective.

Vitamin B_1

Vitamin B_1 (thiamin) is essential for normal nerve function and the production of energy within muscle cells. Diminished sensitivity to pain and temperature and an inability to detect vibrations are indicators of vitamin B_1 deficiency. You may also experience cramping of your calves at night, slight swelling, constipation, and fatigue. B_1 is needed for the body to produce adequate amounts of thyroid hormones (for more on this topic, see "Organ Dysfunction and Disease" in chapter 6). Abuse of alcohol reduces absorption of vitamin B_1, and liver disease will further reduce absorption. Antacids, the tannins in black tea, or a magnesium deficiency can also prevent the absorption. Because vitamin B_1 is water soluble, it will be excreted too rapidly if you're taking diuretics or drinking an excessive amount of water. Vitamin B_1 can be destroyed by processing foods, and by heating them to temperatures above 212°F (100°C).

Self-help technique: Get enough vitamin B_1. Good food sources include lean pork, kidney, liver, beef, eggs, fish, beans, nuts, and some whole grain cereals, if the hull and germ are present.

Vitamin B_6

Vitamin B_6 (pyridoxine) is important for nerve function, energy metabolism, amino acid metabolism, and synthesis of neurotransmitters, including norepinephrine and serotonin, which strongly influence pain perception. Deficiency of B_6 results in anemia, reduced absorption and storage of B_{12}, increased excretion of vitamin C, and blocked synthesis of niacin. It can also lead to a hormonal imbalance. Deficiency of B_6 will manifest as symptoms of deficiency of one of the other B vitamins, since B_6 is needed for all of the others to perform their functions. The need for B_6 increases with age and with eating a high proportion of protein. Tropical sprue (a malabsorption disease) and alcohol use interfere with the body's uptake of B_6. Use of oral contraceptives increases your requirement for B_6 and leads to impaired glucose tolerance (a prediabetic condition). This can lead to depression if you don't supplement with B_6, particularly if you already have a history of depression. Corticosteroid use, excessive alcohol consumption, pregnancy and lactation, antituberculosis drugs, uremia, and hyperthyroidism also increase the need for B_6.

Self-help technique: Get enough vitamin B_6. Good food sources include liver, kidney, chicken (white meat), halibut, tuna, English walnuts, soybean flour, navy beans, bananas, and avocados, but remember that the forms of B_6 found in animal sources are less susceptible to loss due to cooking or preserving than the main form found in plants. There is also some B_6 present in yeast, lean beef, egg yolks, and whole wheat.

Vitamin B_{12}

Vitamin B_{12} (cyanocobalamin) must be taken together with folic acid in order for the body to form red blood cells and rapidly dividing cells such as those found in the gastrointestinal tract, and for the synthesis of fatty acids used in the formation of parts of certain nerve fibers. B_{12} is also needed for metabolism of both fats and carbohydrates. A deficiency can result in pernicious anemia, a condition that reduces the amount of oxygen available to all of your tissues, including muscles and their trigger points, adding to the cycle of dysfunction and increasing pain. A deficiency of B_{12} may also cause nonspecific depression (depression that isn't temporary and isn't due to a specific event), fatigue, an exaggerated startle reaction to noise or touch, and an increased susceptibility to trigger points. Several drugs may impair the absorption of B_{12}, as can megadoses of vitamin C taken for long periods.

Self-help technique: Get enough vitamin B_{12}. Animal products and brewer's yeast grown on a special substrate are the only food sources of vitamin B_{12}. Strict vegetarians must supplement with this vitamin.

Folate

Folate, also known as folic acid when in the synthetic form, is another member of the B complex. A folate deficiency can cause you to be fatigued easily, sleep poorly, or feel discouraged and depressed. It can also cause restless legs syndrome, diffuse muscular pain, diarrhea, or a loss of sensation in your extremities. You may feel cold frequently and have a slightly lower basal body temperature than the normal 98.6°F (37°C). It can also lead to megaloblastic anemia, a condition where the red blood cells are larger than normal, most often due to a deficiency of folate and/or vitamin B_{12}.

In the United States, studies have shown that at least 15 percent of Caucasians are deficient in folate, while at least 30 percent of African-Americans and Latinos are deficient. Part of the problem is that 50 to 95 percent of the folate content of foods may be destroyed during processing and preparation, so even if your diet is rich in foods that are sources of folate, you may not be receiving the benefit (Simons, Travell, and Simons 1999).

Folate is converted into its active form in the digestive system, but this conversion is inhibited by peas, beans, and acidic foods, so eat these separately from your folic acid sources. Those at greatest risk for folate deficiency are the elderly and those who have a bowel disorder, are pregnant or lactating, or use drugs and alcohol regularly. Certain medications deplete folic acid, such as anti-inflammatories (including aspirin), diuretics, estrogens (as in birth control pills and estrogen-based hormone replacement therapy), and anticonvulsants.

Self-help technique: Get enough folate. The best food sources are green leafy vegetables, brewer's yeast, organ meat, fruit, and lightly cooked vegetables such as broccoli and asparagus. As with ascorbic acid (vitamin C), don't take folic acid supplements together with antacids. Also, you must have adequate levels of B_{12} in order to absorb folic acid, and supplementing with only one of these can mask a severe deficiency in the other.

Minerals

Calcium, magnesium, potassium, and iron are needed for proper muscle function. Iron is required for transporting oxygen to the muscle fibers. Calcium is essential for releasing acetylcholine at the nerve terminals, and both calcium and magnesium are needed in order for muscle fibers to contract. Potassium is needed to quickly get muscle fibers ready for their next contraction, and a deficiency may cause muscle soreness during exercise or other physical activity. Deficiency of any of these minerals increases the irritability of trigger points. Calcium, magnesium, and potassium should be taken together, because an increase in one can deplete the others.

Salt is another important mineral. Don't entirely eliminate it from your diet, especially if you sweat. You do need some salt in your diet, unless you have been instructed otherwise by your doctor for certain medical conditions. Inadequate levels of sodium, calcium, magnesium, or potassium can lead to muscle cramping.

Calcium

Tums or other antacids can't substitute for calcium supplements, because they neutralize stomach acid, which is needed for the uptake of calcium. If you must take an antacid, take your calcium-magnesium supplement several hours before or afterward to maximize your absorption. Vitamin D$_3$ is needed for calcium uptake. It is especially important to take calcium for at least a few years prior to menopause to help prevent osteoporosis.

Calcium channel blockers prescribed for high blood pressure inhibit the uptake of calcium into the sarcoplasmic reticulum of vascular smooth muscles and cardiac muscles. Since this is probably also true for skeletal muscles, calcium channel blockers are likely to aggravate trigger points and make them more difficult to treat. If you're taking calcium channel blockers, ask your doctor whether you can switch to a different medication. Consider treating the underlying causes of your high blood pressure with acupuncture, dietary changes, exercise, or whatever is appropriate to your particular set of circumstances.

Self-help technique: Get enough calcium. Good food sources include salmon, sardines, other seafood, green leafy vegetables, almonds, asparagus, blackstrap molasses, brewer's yeast, broccoli, cabbage, carob, collard greens, dandelion greens, figs, filberts, kale, kelp, mustard greens, oats, parsley, prunes, sesame seeds, tofu, and turnip greens. Dairy products and whey are also good sources, but they're contraindicated if you have fibromyalgia or a "damp-type condition" as diagnosed by traditional Chinese medicine.

Magnesium

If you have a healthy diet, you're probably getting enough magnesium; any deficiency is probably due to malabsorption, kidney disease, or fluid and electrolyte loss. Magnesium is depleted after strenuous physical exercise, but reasonable amounts of exercise coupled with an adequate intake of magnesium will improve the efficiency of cellular metabolism and improve your cardiorespiratory performance. Consumption of alcohol, use of diuretics, chronic diarrhea, or consumption of fluoride or high amounts of zinc and vitamin D increase the body's need for magnesium.

Self-help technique: Get enough magnesium. Magnesium is found in most foods, especially meat, fish and other seafood, apples, apricots, avocados, bananas, blackstrap molasses, brewer's yeast, brown rice, figs, garlic, kelp, lima beans, millet, nuts, peaches, black-eyed peas, sesame seeds, tofu, green leafy vegetables, wheat, and whole grains. Dairy products are also good sources, but they're contraindicated if you have fibromyalgia or a "damp-type condition" as diagnosed by traditional Chinese medicine. If you are an athlete, you will probably want to take additional magnesium supplements.

Potassium

A diet high in fats, refined sugars, and salt causes potassium deficiency, as does the use of laxatives and some diuretics. Diarrhea will also deplete potassium. If you experience urinary frequency, particularly if your urine is clear rather than light yellow, try taking potassium. Frequent urination causes potassium deficiency, and because potassium deficiency may, in turn, cause frequent urination, a self-perpetuating cycle can ensue.

Self-help technique: Get enough potassium. Good food sources include fruit (especially bananas and citrus fruits), potatoes, green leafy vegetables, wheat germ, beans, lentils, nuts, dates, and prunes.

Iron

Iron deficiency, which can lead to anemia, is usually caused by excessive blood loss from heavy menses, hemorrhoids, intestinal bleeding, donating blood too often, or ulcers. Iron deficiency can also be caused by a long-term illness, prolonged use of antacids, poor digestion, excessive consumption of coffee or black tea, or the chronic use of NSAIDs (nonsteroidal anti-inflammatory drugs, such as ibuprofen). Early symptoms of iron deficiency include fatigue, reduced endurance, and an inability to stay warm when exposed to a moderately cold environment. Between 9 and 11 percent of menstruating females in the United States are iron deficient, and the worldwide prevalence is about 15 percent (Simons, Travell, and Simons 1999).

If you believe you suffer from an iron deficiency, see your doctor. You shouldn't take iron supplements unless prescribed, other than what is found in a multivitamin or multimineral, because there are health risks associated with taking too much iron. Also, don't take an iron supplement if you have an infection or cancer. The body stores it in order to withhold it from bacteria, and in the case of cancer, it may suppress the cancer-killing function of certain cells.

Self-help technique: Get enough iron—but not too much. Iron is best absorbed with vitamin C. For most people, food sources are adequate for improving iron levels. Good sources include eggs, fish, liver, meat, poultry, green leafy vegetables, whole grains, almonds, avocados, beets, blackstrap molasses, brewer's yeast, dates, egg yolks, kelp, kidney and lima beans, lentils, millet, parsley, peaches, pears, prunes, pumpkin, raisins, sesame seeds, and soybeans. Calcium in milk and other dairy products, or a calcium supplement, can impair absorption of iron, so you should take calcium supplements at a different time than iron supplements.

Water

It's important to drink enough water, because water is the lubricating fluid of your body. Would you drive your car without oil in it? Dehydration is especially common among people who take diuretic medications or drink a lot of coffee or other beverages with diuretic qualities. Don't drink distilled water or rainwater, because you need the minerals found in nondistilled water. If you drink bottled water, know the source of the water to make sure it's not distilled or the minerals otherwise removed. This industry currently isn't regulated, so you may need to do some research on the company.

Self-help technique: Drink enough water. Drink about two quarts of water per day, and more if you have a larger body mass or sweat a lot. Here's a general rule of thumb for people weighing more than 100 pounds: divide your body weight by two, and drink that number of ounces each day. So if you weigh 140 pounds, you should be drinking seventy ounces. Drink at least one extra quart per day if it is very hot out, and drink extra water during and immediately after a workout. Drinking *too* much water is not advisable, since you can deplete vitamin B_1 (thiamin) and other water-soluble vitamins. Also, room-temperature water is better than cold; if you drink something cold, your stomach has to expend energy to warm it up, so it taxes your digestive system.

Improper Diet

Eating foods that aggravate trigger points is a common and significant perpetuating factor. Depending on your constitution, health conditions, and any food allergies, avoiding certain foods can help enormously in relieving your pain.

Plan on avoiding the foods and substances indicated below for at least two months, in conjunction with receiving acupuncture treatments and/or taking herbs and other supplements, in order to determine whether eliminating the specific item is helpful. Many people will stop consuming a food or other substance for just a short while, perhaps only a week, then decide it hasn't made a difference and start consuming those substances again. Or the foods, beverages, or other substances may be so important to them that they'd rather have pain and other medical conditions than give the substances up. Reaching a conclusion after only a short trial period is one way to justify continuing to consume something that causes you problems.

Foods and Drinks to Avoid

You may be reluctant to give up a favorite food or beverage. However, I suggest you read this section and consider that the listed items could be at least part of the cause of your pain. Then you can at least make an informed decision about how committed you are to getting rid of your pain.

Caffeine

Caffeine causes a persistent contracture of muscle fibers (sometimes referred to as "caffeine rigor") and increases muscle tension and trigger point irritability, leading to an increase in pain. It causes excessive amounts of calcium to be released from the sarcoplasmic reticulum and interferes with the rebinding of calcium ions by the sarcoplasmic reticulum. Doctors Travell and Simons (1983) found that caffeine in excess of 150 mg daily (more than two eight-ounce cups of regular coffee) would lead to caffeine rigor. I suspect for some people it could be even less. In assessing your daily intake, be sure to count any caffeine in tea, sodas, and other beverages, and in any drugs you may be taking, and remember that espresso and similar drinks have more concentrated amounts of caffeine.

Alcohol, Tobacco, and Marijuana

Alcohol aggravates trigger points by decreasing serum and tissue levels of folate. It increases the body's need for vitamin C while decreasing the body's ability to absorb it. Tobacco also increases the need for vitamin C.

In traditional Chinese medicine, caffeine and alcohol are said to be very "qi stagnating." The ancient concept of qi is not easily translatable into Western medical terminology. It is thought that qi is energy that flows through fourteen main "meridians" and connecting vessels that go to all parts of the body. Qi moves the blood and lymph fluids. When the flow of qi is blocked (stagnation), pain and disease result. Based on today's understanding of body processes, some think that qi refers to the biochemical processes in living creatures—the combination of electrical impulses, neurotransmitters, hormones, body fluids, and cellular metabolism that allow us to be living, breathing creatures. As you read in chapter 1, trigger points form when your fluids aren't moving well, cellular metabolism isn't working properly, and neurotransmitters aren't operating normally, which supports that particular concept of qi, and the idea of pain resulting from qi stagnation.

Marijuana is also very stagnating, and it stays in your system for about three months after smoking it. Stagnation is one cause of pain; therefore, using any of these substances will increase your pain level.

Food Allergies

Exposure to both environmental and food-related allergens causes the body to release histamines, which perpetuates trigger points and makes them harder to treat. Avoiding allergenic foods can be challenging when you're dining out, traveling, or eating at someone else's home. Whenever it's feasible, bring along something you can eat so you'll have an alternative.

Self-help technique: Do a self-test for food allergens. There are a few methods of testing for food allergens. One of the best ways is an elimination diet, where you eliminate all suspect foods, then add them back in one at a time, and then rotate foods. You can find instructions for this in *Prescription for Nutritional Healing* (Balch and Balch 2000), under "Allergies." However, most people aren't willing to take this approach, as it requires you to be very disciplined about your diet and keep a careful food diary for a month. As an alternative, *Prescription for Nutritional Healing* offers a quick test. After sitting and relaxing for a few minutes, take your pulse rate for one minute, and then eat the food you are testing. Keep still for fifteen to twenty minutes and take your pulse again. If your pulse rate has increased more than ten beats per minute, eliminate this food from your diet for one month, then retest. Another option is a blood test for food allergens, offered by naturopaths and some other practitioners.

Conclusion

Improving your nutrition, changing your diet, and avoiding detrimental foods, beverages, and inhaled substances will likely take some time, but you can start by taking a multivitamin and multimineral supplement and drinking enough water. As you identify which foods you need to avoid, start replacing them with foods high in the vitamins and minerals discussed in this chapter. Be sure you are getting enough protein.

The next chapter covers the remaining perpetuating factors that are most likely to cause and perpetuate trigger points, including emotional factors, sleep problems, acute and chronic infections, hormonal imbalances, and organ dysfunction and disease.

Chapter 6

Other Perpetuating Factors

Several other factors that can perpetuate trigger points are worth mentioning, since they may play an important role in your lower leg, knee, ankle, or foot pain. Emotional factors such as anxiety and depression, sleep problems, acute and chronic infections, hormonal imbalances, and organ dysfunction and disease can all be involved in the formation and perpetuation of trigger points. Laboratory tests are required to diagnose some of these conditions, so you'll probably need to work with a doctor to determine whether those factors are involved in causing your trigger points.

Emotional Factors

Emotional factors can contribute greatly to causing and perpetuating pain—and many other health conditions as well. As you may recall from chapter 1, while prolonged exposure to both emotional and physical stressors can lead to central nervous system sensitization and subsequently cause pain, conversely prolonged pain can also lead to central nervous system sensitization, leading to emotional and physical stress (Niddam 2009). Also remember that once the central nervous system is sensitized, pain can be more easily triggered by lower levels of physical and emotional stressors and be more intense and last longer (Latremoliere and Woolf 2009).

While it's encouraging that modern medicine has accepted the role of emotional factors, all too often people are dismissed by their doctors as "just being under stress." The appointment ends and their physical symptoms are neither assessed nor addressed. This is particularly true when it comes to pain and depression. If you're in pain long enough, of course you'll begin to feel fatigued, depressed, and anxious. The converse is also true: if you're depressed, anxious, and fatigued long enough, you'll probably develop pain. It's important to recognize the role of stress and emotional factors as both a cause of illness and a result of illness, and to address them just as you would any other factor.

Depression

If you experience an unusual desire to be alone, a loss of interest in your favorite activities, and a decrease in job performance, and are neglecting your appearance and hygiene, you may be suffering from more than a mild and temporary situation-dependent depression. Clinical symptoms of depression are insomnia, loss of appetite, weight loss, impotence or decreased libido, blurred vision, a sad mood, thoughts of suicide or death, an inability to concentrate, poor memory, indecision, mumbled speech, and negative reactions to suggestions. There can certainly be other reasons for some of these symptoms, and no single symptom is indicative of depression. It is the number and combination of symptoms that leads to a diagnosis of clinical depression. However, if you are having thoughts of suicide or self-harm for any reason, it is imperative that you seek help immediately.

Depression lowers your pain threshold, increases the amount of pain you feel, and adversely affects your response to trigger point therapy. There are many approaches to treating depression (see below), including medications. While antidepressants may help with the acute symptoms, many of them have side effects. Plus, some medications can exacerbate the underlying condition causing the symptoms, so a vicious cycle ensues.

Anxiety

If you are extremely anxious, chances are you're holding tension in at least some of your muscles and developing trigger points as a result. Holding tension in your back, shoulders, and gluteal muscles affects your legs both indirectly through central sensitization and directly through referral patterns that extend into your legs.

Self-Help Technique: Get help for emotional factors. If you are depressed or anxious, you need to address this in order to speed your recovery from pain. Unfortunately people suffering from severe depression, anxiety, chronic fatigue, or extreme pain often don't have the energy to participate in their own healing. You may have difficulty summoning the energy to cook healthy foods or even get out of bed, and you may not be able to manage to do even mild forms of exercise, such as walking—the very things that would help you start to feel better. You may have a hard time making it to appointments with a counselor or health care practitioner. If this describes you, you need to do whatever you can to get to the point where you can start taking better care of yourself. This may mean taking homeopathic remedies, receiving acupuncture treatments or counseling, or doing the self-help techniques in this book. You may need to take antidepressants or pain relievers for a while until you feel well enough to start using the above suggestions. Just doing one of these things will help get you started in the right direction and improve your energy and outlook.

One of the things I like most about Oriental medicine and homeopathy is that both assume you can't separate the physical body from the emotions. These systems of healing consider both physical and emotional symptoms in developing a diagnosis, and both types of symptoms are treated simultaneously. With acupuncture, there are no side effects and response is usually rapid. With both homeopathy and herbs, the wrong prescription or dosage can have side effects, just as with allopathic prescription drugs, so it is important to consult with a trained professional. Detailed recommendations for treating either depression or anxiety are beyond the scope of this book, but many excellent self-help books on the topic are available. Also see the section on the thyroid in "Organ Dysfunction and Disease" later in this chapter, since thyroid problems can be an undiagnosed cause of depression.

Self-help technique: Get enough exercise. Exercise increases levels of serotonin, a neurotransmitter believed to play an important role in many body functions, including mood regulation. Walking and deep breathing are great for relieving tension, anxiety, and depression. Even walking ten minutes per day can be extremely beneficial, especially if you can walk outside.

Self-help technique: Notice when you're tensing—and relax! Notice whether you're hiking your shoulders up or tightening muscles, particularly when you're under stress. Take a minute to mentally assess your body, noticing where you're holding tension. Whenever you come to an area that's tense, take a deep breath and consciously relax the area as you exhale. Do this several times each day. You will need to retrain yourself to break the habit of holding tension in certain areas.

Sleep Problems

Sleep disorders, interrupted sleep, and insufficient sleep can all perpetuate trigger points, and both the trigger points themselves and the lack of sleep can contribute to pain. The first step in solving this problem is to consider whether you had sleep problems before your lower leg, knee, ankle, or foot pain started. If you did, then the underlying factors responsible for your sleep problems must be addressed.

Self-help technique: Treat your pain. If pain disturbs you at night, use the self-treatments described in part III to work on your trigger points when you're awakened by pain. Hopefully this will allow you to fall back to sleep once your pain abates. If you're using a ball for self-treatment, as described in part III, you don't fall asleep on the ball, since doing so will cut off the circulation for too long and make the trigger points worse.

Self-help technique: Check your environment. Be sure you aren't sleeping poorly due to being too warm or too cold. Fortunately this is relatively easy to address. If noise is waking you, try wearing earplugs. My favorite type is Mack's Pillow Soft silicone earplugs. Computer use or possibly watching TV in the evening can overstimulate the brain and make it hard to fall asleep and sleep restfully.

Make sure you aren't being exposed to allergens at night. Many people are allergic to dust mites, which live in bedding, among other places. An inexpensive solution is to use soft vinyl covers over your pillows and mattress. If you have a down comforter or pillow, you may be allergic to the feathers even if you aren't exhibiting classic allergy symptoms, such as sneezing and itchy eyes. Or it may be that your mattress is worn out, or that your mattress or pillows are inappropriate for your body. See "Misfitting Furniture" in chapter 4 for more information and recommendations.

Self-help technique: Try acupuncture, herbs, or other supplements. Acupuncture and Chinese herbs may be helpful, especially if your mind is overactive, you sleep lightly and wake frequently, you wake up early and can't fall back to sleep, you have vivid and disturbing dreams, or you're menopausal. If urinary frequency is disturbing your sleep, try acupuncture, herbs, and increasing your potassium intake. If you have problems falling asleep, try improving your diet, taking supplements, and drinking enough water—but don't drink too much just before bedtime! Taking a calcium-magnesium supplement before bedtime can be especially helpful, particularly if you are experiencing calf cramps.

Self-help technique: Eliminate caffeine & alcohol. Caffeine and alcohol will disturb your sleep or make you sleep more lightly, in addition to aggravating trigger points (see chapter 5). Even if you only drink caffeine in the morning, it can still disrupt your nighttime sleep patterns. If you choose to give up caffeine, you may experience various withdrawal symptoms, and the first few days can be difficult. It will take about two weeks before your energy starts to even out and you feel like you don't need caffeine to get going in the morning.

Self-help technique: Rest & relax more. If you are continually under stress, or if you're pushing yourself too hard and push through fatigue instead of resting or taking a nap, your adrenal glands will excrete excessive amounts of adrenaline, which can interfere with sleep. A naturopathic doctor can administer a saliva test for adrenal function. Try breathing deeply until you fall asleep.

Acute or Chronic Infections

Infections are trigger point perpetuators that are often overlooked. If you have an infection that is affecting your legs, such as the *neuralgia* (pain along the course of a nerve) of genital herpes, it is extremely important to eliminate or manage the infection in order to get relief from the pain.

Acute Infections

Try to head off acute illnesses, such as colds and flu, at the first sign in order to avoid perpetuating trigger points. This is particularly important if you have fibromyalgia, sinusitis, asthma, or recurrent infections, since your trigger points will be activated by illness. Getting sick can set you back by months in your treatment and healing.

Self-help technique: Don't get sick. With lifestyle modifications and preventive care, it is possible to reduce your incidence of illness. When you start to get sick, take echinacea, the Chinese herbal formulas Gan Mao Ling or Yin Chiao, and/or homeopathic remedies as appropriate, such as Oscillococcinum for flu. Keep these herbs and remedies on hand at home so you can take them as soon as you notice the first signs of illness. Once you're past the initial stage of illness, the herbs or remedies you need will depend on your particular set of symptoms, so you may need to consult with a practitioner.

Chronic Infections

Chronic infections such as sinus infections, urinary tract infections, and herpes simplex (cold sores, genital herpes, or shingles) will perpetuate trigger points, so you need to resolve or manage chronic infections to obtain lasting relief from lower leg, knee, ankle, or foot pain, and from trigger points in general.

With both sinus infections and urinary tract infections, antibiotics often don't kill all of the pathogens, and you end up with lingering, recurrent infections. However, antibiotics have the advantage of working quickly, so I often recommend combining antibiotics with other treatments, such as acupuncture, herbs, and homeopathic remedies. This will knock the infection out as quickly and completely as possible, and help prevent it from becoming a chronic problem. Urinary tract infections must be dealt with promptly. You can use over-the-counter allopathic drugs, Chinese herbs, or cranberry extract or juice (don't use sweetened juice), but if your symptoms don't improve right away, you need to see your doctor. Urinary tract infections can turn into life-threatening kidney infections.

A variety of supplements, herbs, and pharmaceutical drugs are used to treat recurrent herpes infections, and some will work better than others for you. If you have recurrent outbreaks, you need to figure out what is impairing your immune system, such as allergies or emotional stress. Sometimes a herpes outbreak is the first sign that your body is fighting an acute illness. This can be a signal to you to take the remedies mentioned above.

Parasitic Infections

The fish tapeworm, giardia, and the amoeba are the parasites most likely to perpetuate trigger points. The fish tapeworm and giardia both scar the lining of the intestines and impair your ability to absorb nutrients, and they also consume vitamin B_{12}. Amoeba can produce toxins that are passed from the intestines into the body. Fish tapeworms can be present in raw fish. Giardia is most often associated with drinking untreated water from streams, but it can also be passed by an infected person who doesn't wash their hands after a bowel movement, particularly if they are preparing food or have some other hand-to-mouth contact.

If you have chronic diarrhea, it is worth testing for parasites. However, such tests can be costly, and different tests are required to rule out different parasites. A cheaper alternative is to treat a suspected parasitic infection with herbs like grapefruit seed extract or pulsatilla (a Chinese herb) and see if your symptoms improve. However, if you have blood in your stools, you should see your doctor immediately to rule out serious conditions.

Many people report feeling much better on an anticandida diet, and in any case it is a pretty healthy way to eat. The basics of the diet are to avoid sugar in all its forms, simple and processed carbohydrates, fermented foods, yeast, mushrooms, and certain cheeses. There are many herbal products on the market for eliminating candida, including grapefruit seed extract, oil of oregano, echinacea, pulsatilla, and a variety of formulas. Since most of these will also kill off your beneficial intestinal flora, you need to use a good multiacidophilus supplement after treatment, as you would after taking any antibiotic.

Organ Dysfunction and Disease

Organ dysfunction and disease, such as hypothyroidism, hypometabolism, hypoglycemia, diabetes, and gout, can cause and perpetuate trigger points. Even though these are among the more challenging perpetuating factors to address, treating them is absolutely essential for pain relief.

Thyroid

Both subclinical hypothyroidism (also known as hypometabolism or thyroid inadequacy) and hypothyroidism will cause and perpetuate trigger points. People who have a low-functioning thyroid gland may experience early-morning stiffness and pain and weakness of the shoulder girdle. Symptoms of both subclinical hypothyroidism and hypothyroidism include intolerance to cold (and sometimes heat), cold hands and feet, muscle aches and pains (especially with cold, rainy weather), constipation, menstrual problems, weight gain, dry skin, fatigue, and lethargy. Muscles feel rather hard to the touch, and even if people with hypothyroidism take a thyroid supplement, I've noticed they are still somewhat prone to trigger points, probably because it's hard to fine-tune the dosage to the exact amount the person's body would produce if the thyroid gland were healthy.

Some studies report that as many as 17 percent of women and 7 percent of men have subclinical hypothyroidism (Simons, Travell, and Simons 1999). Contrary to the usual symptoms, some people with subclinical hypothyroidism may be thin, nervous, and hyperactive, and in these cases practitioners may not consider the possibility of hypometabolism.

People with low thyroid function may be low in vitamin B_1 (thiamin). Before starting on thyroid medication, try supplementing with B_1 to see if that corrects your thyroid hormone levels. If you are already on thyroid medication and you start taking B_1, you may develop symptoms of hyperthyroidism, in which case your medication dosage must be adjusted. If you are low in B_1 when you start taking thyroid medication, you may develop symptoms of acute B_1 deficiency, which may be misinterpreted as an intolerance to the medication. After the B_1 deficiency is corrected, you will likely tolerate the medication. You need to supplement with B_1 prior to and during thyroid hormone therapy to avoid a deficiency. Total body potassium is low in hypothyroidism and high in hyperthyroidism, so you may need to adjust your potassium intake as well.

Smoking impairs the action of thyroid hormones and will make any related symptoms worse. Several pharmaceutical drugs can also affect thyroid hormone levels, such as lithium, anticonvulsants, glucocorticoid steroids, and drugs that contain iodine. If you've been diagnosed with hypothyroidism and are taking other medications, consult with your doctor or pharmacist to see whether any of your medications could be causing the problem.

Self-help technique: Test your thyroid function at home. A simple home test to check your thyroid function is to measure your basal body temperature. Place a thermometer in your armpit for ten minutes upon waking and before getting out of bed. Normal underarm temperature for men and postmenopausal women is 98°F (36.7°C). For premenopausal women, it's 97.5°F (36.4°C) prior to ovulation and 98.5°F (36.9°C) after ovulation. If your temperature is lower than this, consult with your doctor.

Self-help technique: Get the right tests. Often doctors initially test only TSH (thyroid stimulating hormone) levels. The results may still be normal if you have subclinical hypothyroidism rather than clinical hypothyroidism. A radioimmunoassay measures levels of two specific thyroid hormones—T3 and T4—and gives a more complete picture of your thyroid function. If you are depressed, insist that your thyroid levels be tested before you start taking antidepressant medication. If thyroid dysfunction is responsible for your depression, correcting it may resolve the depression, allowing you to avoid antidepressants and their many side effects. I've had more than one patient (especially men) whose hypothyroidism was discovered only after they had been medicated with antidepressants for some time.

Hypoglycemia

Hypoglycemia is an abnormally low level of glucose in the blood. This is most often related to diabetes, but there are several other, less common possible causes. A hypoglycemic reaction when a meal is delayed (fasting hypoglycemia) usually indicates a problem with the liver, adrenal glands, or pituitary gland. Missing or delaying a meal won't cause hypoglycemia in a healthy person. Onset of hypoglycemia after a meal (reactive hypoglycemia) usually occurs two to three hours after eating a meal rich in carbohydrates and is most likely to occur when you are under a lot of stress. You need to identify the causes and address them if possible.

If you've been diagnosed with hypoglycemia, you probably know the cause and whether it is reactive or fasting hypoglycemia. The important thing to know is that both types cause and perpetuate trigger points and make trigger points more difficult to treat. Symptoms of both types are sweating, trembling and shakiness, increased heart rate, and anxiety. If allowed to progress, symptoms of severe hypoglycemia can include visual disturbances, restlessness, and impaired speech and thinking. Avoid all caffeine, alcohol, and tobacco (even secondhand smoke). Normally the liver converts the body's stored carbohydrates into glucose when blood glucose levels drop, and this helps avoid or slow down a hypoglycemic reaction. When you ingest alcohol, caffeine, or tobacco, your liver considers detoxifying your bloodstream the highest priority and will not put more glucose into the bloodstream until it is done, resulting in a hypoglycemic reaction.

Self-help technique: Eat small, frequent meals. Symptoms of hypoglycemia will be relieved by eating smaller, more frequent meals with fewer carbohydrates, more protein, and some fat. If you are waking up with pain or are having trouble sleeping, eating a small snack or drinking a little juice before you go to bed may help. Also, acupuncture is quite successful in stabilizing blood sugar.

Type II Diabetes and Obesity

Diabetes and obesity are extremely hard on your body in general, and on your legs and feet in particular. Often medical practitioners don't want to point this out; I know that I'm hesitant to say, "You need to lose weight," both being reluctant to state the obvious and being afraid I'll make someone feel worse about themselves than they may already feel. It's not like someone doesn't know they are overweight.

Food addictions are the toughest ones to "recover" from. After all, you can't just "quit cold turkey" like you can with other addictions. You still have to eat. I have complete and total sympathy and empathy with you if you're struggling with your weight. I know it's not as simple as someone saying to you, "Just eat less." But I'm going to lay out the facts for you, along with some helpful suggestions.

Diabetes

Diabetes can cause problems in a number of ways. Your compromised circulatory system doesn't bring enough oxygen, nutrients, and natural wound-fighting blood cells to your legs. You lose sensation in your legs, which makes you unable to detect when you are being injured either acutely or by chronic microtrauma. The subsequent damage to your tissues results in foot ulcers that the body can't heal. The lack of adequate circulation leads to uncontrollable infections and gangrene. Eventually your leg may need to be amputated if the disease progresses. Diabetes is a leading cause of death and skyrocketing medical costs, and—more often than not—is preventable. See your health care provider for self-help techniques that are appropriate for your situation. If you have reduced sensation in your legs and feet, be careful when applying pressure with the techniques found in this book; err on the side of pressing too lightly.

Obesity

If you are overweight or obese, you are overloading the bones, joints, ligaments, and tendons of your legs and feet. A sedentary lifestyle causes bone loss and atrophied muscles, which then aren't able to protect the joints. If you also have diabetes and other diseases that reduce circulation, they can slow or stop healing. *Losing weight is one of the most effective early interventions for treating leg and foot problems*, by decreasing the load on the structures, and by reducing the chronic inflammation linked with excessive fat (adipose) tissue.

Self-help technique: Eat better and get mild to moderate amounts of exercise. Establishing healthy eating habits, as opposed to fad diets, is crucial to long-term, gradual weight loss and better nutrition. In addition to improving your diet, you should exercise. Exercising in a pool is preferable initially, since it doesn't place a large strain on your lower limbs. Even if you can walk short distances daily, it will speed up your metabolism and make you feel better, in addition to helping you lose weight. You may wish to use two hiking or ski poles, which will help you keep your balance and provide an upper body work-out as well. You may be able to use a stationary bike even if you can't walk. Find an "exercise buddy" to help keep you on track. If calf and foot pain are keeping you from exercising, use the techniques found in this book so you can get to the point where you can get some form of exercise.

If emotional eating is an issue, find support. Many of my patients have had success with Weight Watchers and Overeaters Anonymous, where they have a supportive atmosphere coupled with a focus on changing habits, as opposed to going on fad diets. There are a lot of resources available, if you should choose to use them. Do not undergo any drastic weight loss program or an increase in exercise without the supervision of a qualified practitioner. Whatever you choose to do, set small, attainable goals so you can experience successes. Setting unreasonable goals sets you up for failure and a self-sabotaging return to your previous eating and exercise habits.

Gout

Gout is a disease characterized by high uric acid levels in the blood. It is caused by dietary factors, genetics, or the underexcretion of urate (the salts of uric acid). Monosodium urate (MSU) crystals form and are deposited in joints, tendons, and the surrounding tissues, which then usually causes swelling and intense pain due to an inflammatory reaction. The joint at the base of the big toe is most commonly affected. Gout often occurs in combination with obesity, diabetes, hypertension, insulin resistance, and/or abnormal lipid levels.

Gout will aggravate trigger points and make them difficult to treat. While Doctors Travell and Simons did not speculate in their books as to why gout is a perpetuating factor for trigger points, it is likely that trigger points are caused and perpetuated by the high acid content, in addition to causing a self-perpetuating cycle of pain from central sensitization. (See "Elevated Biochemicals" in chapter 1).

Conclusion

Eliminating perpetuating factors may possibly give you complete relief from pain without any additional treatment. If you don't resolve or avoid perpetuating factors to the extent possible, you may not get more than temporary relief from any form of treatment.

Hopefully you've learned enough about your potential perpetuating factors that even if you choose not to resolve them, you'll be making an informed choice about which you value more: relief from your lower leg, knee, ankle, or foot pain, or continuing to do things that make you feel worse, even if they are within your power to change. You will have more control over some perpetuating factors than others. For example, you may not be able to control whether you have hypothyroidism, but you can take thyroid hormones and supplements and stop smoking. You have also learned how obesity and diabetes can contribute to pain and trigger point formation both directly and indirectly. Much or all of your lower leg, knee, ankle, or foot pain is probably within your control. What are you willing to do to change your life?

The next section will teach you how to work on your own trigger points, how to stretch properly, how to care for your muscles, and what you should avoid doing so that you don't make yourself feel worse.

Part III

TRIGGER POINT SELF-HELP TECHNIQUES

In this section, you'll learn how to relieve your trigger points with self-help techniques. Chapter 7 provides general guidelines on how to do trigger point self-treatments and what to avoid, as well as some do's and don'ts for stretching and conditioning. Chapter 8 helps you determine which trigger points cause your lower limb pain. Each of the remaining chapters covers a muscle or group of muscles that may contain trigger points which can contribute to leg, knee, ankle, or foot pain.

In the muscle chapters, anatomical drawings are provided to help you locate where trigger points are most likely located in the muscle and to see what the muscle looks like. Symptom lists and photographs showing pain referral patterns, and lists of common causes and perpetuating factors for trigger points, will help you determine whether a given trigger point might be causing your pain. These are followed by helpful hints for dealing with those causes. Photographs and written instructions provide guidance on self-treatment of trigger points. Most of the muscle chapters also include stretches. Each muscle chapter will also advise you to check other muscles that may be involved.

Chapter 7

General Guidelines for Self-Treatment

In this chapter, you'll learn how to apply pressure to trigger points and how to stretch and condition muscles properly. I'll also offer general guidelines on caring for your muscles in order to prevent the reactivation of trigger points.

General Guidelines for Applying Pressure During Self-Treatments

Applying pressure on your own trigger points can give you a great deal of relief within the first few weeks, but you must perform the techniques properly. You can expect gradual improvement over a period of days and weeks. Review the following guidelines frequently in the beginning stages of treatment, and then periodically to ensure you are performing the techniques properly.

How Not to Perform Self-Treatments

The most important guideline is this: don't overdo it! Many people think that if some self-treatment feels good, doing it harder, longer, or more often will be even more helpful. But you can actually make yourself worse by doing treatments too frequently or doing them incorrectly.

Don't apply pressure over varicose veins, open wounds, infected areas, herniated or bulging disks, areas affected by phlebitis or thrombophlebitis, or anywhere clots are present or could be present. If you're pregnant, don't apply pressure on your legs.

If your symptoms get worse or you are sore from treatments for more than one day, stop the self-treatments for a few days until your symptoms improve, then resume doing the treatments less frequently and using less pressure to see if you can tolerate them without feeling worse or sore. Chances are you were using too much pressure or holding the points for too long. Review these guidelines if that is the case. If you're seeing a practitioner, they may be able to help you figure out any problems with how you are doing the self-treatments. And if you are sore from a therapist's work, be sure to tell them.

How to Work on Trigger Points

The most important technique for treating trigger points, other than eliminating perpetuating factors, is applying pressure. Use a tennis ball, racquetball, golf ball, dog play ball, or baseball, or use your elbow or hand if instructed to do so for particular muscles. When lying on balls, use only the weight of your body to give you pressure. Don't actively press your back or other body parts onto the balls. The muscle you're working on should be as passive as possible. Use only one ball at a time on your back, not one on each side. If you need to work on your back muscles during the workday, I recommend getting a Backnobber, a large S-shaped gadget for applying pressure, available from the Pressure Positive Company (see Resources) and other sources.

Apply pressure for a minimum of eight seconds (less than that may activate trigger points) and a maximum of one minute (to avoid cutting off the circulation for too long, which could aggravate the trigger point). You can count out the time by saying "one one thousand, two one thousand, three one thousand," and so on. Time yourself first to be sure you are actually counting seconds at the correct speed; don't race to eight as quickly as possible.

The pressure should be somewhat uncomfortable but hurt in a good way. It shouldn't be so painful that you tense up or hold your breath. If you're using a ball and the treatment is too painful, move to a softer surface such as a bed, or pad the surface with a pillow or blanket. Alternatively, try using a smaller or softer ball. You can puncture a tennis ball with a nail to make it softer. If the treatment doesn't produce tenderness at all, keep looking for tender spots or try moving to a harder surface. If you're using a ball for treatment but the trigger point is too tender for you to lie on it at all, try putting the ball in a long sock and leaning against the wall. However, I recommend this only if you can't lie on the ball, since leaning against the wall involves using the very muscles you are trying to work on. You may need to use a combination of surfaces depending on the tenderness of different areas. Over time, as your sensitivity decreases and you're able to work the deeper parts of the muscle, you may need to use a ball that's harder or a different size, or to move to a harder surface. Experiment to find what's effective for you.

If your time is limited, treat one area thoroughly rather than rushing through many areas. If you hurry, you're more likely to aggravate trigger points rather than inactivate them.

If you're using a ball for self-treatment, be careful not to fall asleep on the ball, since doing so will cut off the circulation for too long and make the trigger points worse. When you're fatigued and in pain and suddenly the pain is reduced or gone, it's all too easy to fall asleep on the ball, so don't use this technique in bed unless you're sure that won't happen.

Where to Find Trigger Points

Search the entire muscle for tender points, particularly the points of maximum tenderness, to make sure you find all the potential trigger points. Use the muscle drawings and pictures in the following chapters to make sure you're searching the entire muscle and not just focusing on the most painful spot. Many times a tendon attachment will hurt because the tight muscle is pulling on it, but if you don't work on the entire belly of the muscle, it will keep pulling on the attachment.

If you find trigger points on one side of the body, be sure to work on the same muscles on the other side, but spend more time on the side that's causing your pain. Except for very new one-sided injuries, the same muscle on the opposite side will almost always also be tender with applied pressure, even if it hasn't started causing symptoms yet. For back muscles, loosening one side but not the other can lead to new problems. And sometimes the muscles on the opposite side are actually causing the symptoms, so it's always worthwhile to work on both sides.

Pressure on a trigger point may reproduce the referred pain pattern, but this doesn't always occur. So if you have reason to suspect that a particular muscle is involved, work on it anyway and see if it helps relieve your pain and other symptoms.

Work in the direction of referral. For example, if trigger points in the gluteus minimus muscle are referring pain to your thigh and calf, work on the gluteus minimus muscle first, then the thigh and lower leg.

If treatments seem effective but you get only temporary relief, start searching for trigger points that refer pain or other symptoms to the area you've already located and treated for trigger points. It may be that you have been working on satellite trigger points and need to locate the primary trigger points that are activating the satellite trigger points. You can't resolve satellite trigger points without first addressing the primary trigger points causing them. For example, if you have lower leg pain and you can get only temporary relief by working on the peroneal muscles, consider whether referral from trigger points in the anterior portion of the gluteus minimus muscle are keeping the peroneal trigger points active. In this case, the peroneal muscles contain the satellite trigger points, and the gluteus minimus contains the primary trigger points.

Each muscle chapter contains a list of other muscles that may also be involved (under "Also See"). However, because each person's body is so different, you may need to look through the referral patterns in all of the muscle chapters to determine which other muscles may be involved in your case.

Frequency of Self-Treatments

Most people should work on their muscles one time per day initially. Pick a time when you'll remember to do your self-treatments—perhaps when you wake up, when you watch television, or when you go to bed—and keep your balls where they'll be handy. (Just be careful not to fall asleep on a ball!) If you're sore from self-treatments or your practitioner's treatments, skip a day. If you're seeing a practitioner, don't do self-treatments on the same day you have an appointment.

After a few weeks, you can increase your self-treatments to twice per day as long as you're not getting sore. If a particular activity seems to aggravate your trigger points, try doing self-treatments before and after the activity. If you start getting sore or your symptoms get worse, decrease the frequency.

Take your balls with you on trips, since travel frequently aggravates trigger points. You may even want to keep some balls or a Backnobber at work.

Keep working on the muscle until it is no longer tender, even if your active symptoms have disappeared. Just because a trigger point isn't causing referred pain doesn't mean the trigger point is gone. It has probably just become latent, in which case it could easily be reactivated. If you leave your trigger points untreated or stop treatment too soon, it is more likely that the changes to your nervous system will be long-term or permanent, and that the pain will recur more easily. As your symptoms disappear, you may feel less motivated to do treatments or even forget to do them. Try not to let this happen. But if it does, the important thing is that you will know what to do if symptoms return.

General Guidelines for Stretches and Conditioning

It is very important to distinguish between stretching and conditioning exercises. With stretching, you gently lengthen the muscle fibers, whereas with conditioning exercises you're trying to strengthen the muscle. Doctors Travell and Simons (1983) found that active trigger points benefited from stretching but were usually aggravated by conditioning exercises in the early stages of treatment.

Often people start physical therapy and trigger point therapy at the same time, but this may be counterproductive, as physical therapy usually relies heavily on conditioning exercises unless the physical therapist is familiar with trigger points. In my experience, when the two are done concurrently in the initial stages of treatment, over half the time the person's condition either doesn't improve or actually gets worse. Usually you can start doing conditioning exercises after about two weeks of trigger point treatment and self-help work, but if your trigger points are still very irritable, you will need to wait until your symptoms improve. Meanwhile, learn the stretching exercises in this book. As long as you follow the guidelines, these do not need to be prescribed by a practitioner.

If you aren't sure whether an assigned activity is a stretch or a conditioning exercise, ask your practitioner. Also be sure to tell your practitioner all the activities, exercises, and stretches you're doing, because some of these could be contributing to activating your trigger points. I won't cover guidelines for conditioning exercises in depth here, since they should be prescribed by a practitioner, who can also give you instructions for performing them safely and effectively.

Things to Avoid when Stretching and Conditioning

Avoid stretching when your muscles are tired or cold, and don't bounce on stretches. Friends may recommend conditioning exercises that worked for them, but you are a different person with a different set of symptoms, and you shouldn't do conditioning exercises prescribed for them, just as you wouldn't take their prescribed medications. If a conditioning exercise or stretch is aggravating your symptoms, stop doing it. Consult with your practitioner to determine why it is bothering you and how you should proceed.

When and How to Do Stretches and Conditioning

Do your stretches *after* treating your trigger points. If you have time to do only one thing, do the self-treatments and skip the stretches. Trigger point inactivation followed by stretching is more effective than trigger point inactivation alone, but stretching without prior inactivation can actually increase trigger point sensitivity (Edwards and Knowles 2003).

Stretch slowly, and only to the point of just getting a gentle stretch. Don't force it. If you stretch muscles too hard or too fast, you can aggravate trigger points. Hold each stretch for thirty to sixty seconds. There will be little benefit after thirty seconds, but stretching for longer won't hurt you. You may repeat the stretch after releasing and breathing. For any type of repetitive exercise, breathe and rest between each repetition of the exercise.

If your stretches or conditioning exercises make you sore for more than one day, try again after the soreness has disappeared and reduce the number of repetitions. If you're still sore two days after the exercise or stretch, you may be doing it incorrectly or it might not be the right stretch for you and need to be eliminated or changed (Travell and Simons 1983).

General Guidelines for Muscle Care

In addition to inactivating your trigger points and stretching, you need to take good care of your muscles. This will help prevent reactivation of old trigger points and the development of new ones.

Muscle Awareness

After treatments, gently use the muscle in a normal way, using its full range of motion, but avoid strenuous activities for at least one day or until the trigger points aren't so easily aggravated, whichever is longer. Go slowly and be gentle with yourself.

Rest and take frequent breaks from any given activity, and don't sit for too long in one position. Learn to avoid keeping your muscles in prolonged contractions, where you are holding them tense or using them in a sustained way. To increase blood flow and bring oxygen and nutrients to the muscles, they need to alternately constrict and relax, which normal, fairly frequent movement will accomplish. Notice where you hold tension and practice relaxing that area. Avoid cold drafts.

Lift with your knees bent and your back straight, holding the object you're lifting close to your chest. Don't lift something too heavy—ask for help. Never put the maximum load on a muscle. It's too easy to strain your muscles when you do this.

Exercise Programs

Before doing any type of exercise, warm up adequately. Tight, cold muscles are more prone to injury. As always, as with any exercise, avoid positions or activities that aggravate any medical condition. Swimming is generally a good exercise, and bicycling is easier on the body than running, but in both cases you must take care to avoid straining your trapezius and neck muscles. Any bike that allows you to sit more upright, such as a recumbent or stationary bicycle, is preferable to those that require you to lean over the handlebars.

When starting an exercise program, underestimate what you will be able to do, and err on the side of caution. Many people believe in the adage "no pain, no gain" and think that pushing through the pain will make them stronger. But this just aggravates existing problems and makes them harder to treat. Exercise should be comfortable. Alternate running with walking or, when lifting weights, rest between repetitions and use weights that aren't too heavy. If you tend to overdo things, you need to back off on your activities, then add them back in slowly with the guidance of your practitioner. Returning to activities too soon or doing them excessively will quickly erode your progress.

Gradually increase the duration, rate, and effort of any exercises in small increments that don't cause soreness or trigger point activation. Mild to moderate aerobic exercise is good for overall health and for preventing the recurrence of muscular problems. It's also great for reducing stress. People who exercise regularly are less likely to develop trigger points than those who exercise occasionally and overdo it. Just don't overdo it!

Conclusion

In this chapter, you've learned the basics of trigger point self-treatments, along with what to avoid when doing self-treatments. You've also learned some of the basics about how to stretch, and how to take care of your muscles to prevent reactivation of trigger points and the formation of new trigger points. The most important thing to remember is what not to do: don't overdo trigger point treatments, stretching, conditioning, or exercise programs. Review the guidelines in this chapter frequently in the beginning stages of treatment, and then review them periodically thereafter to ensure that you are performing the techniques properly.

The next chapter will help you identify which muscles may be causing your leg, knee, ankle, or foot pain and other symptoms. It will also offer guidance on recording your symptoms and tracking your progress.

Chapter 8

Which Muscles Are Causing My Pain?

The last chapter taught you *how* to treat trigger points; this chapter helps you find *where to look* for trigger points that are causing your particular set of symptoms.

Pain Map

To figure out which muscles to work on first, look at the Pain Map on page 76. Find the area(s) where you feel your pain, and read the chapters listed by number. The muscles in the menus are listed in order from top to bottom of the most common muscles to refer pain to an area, but it may be different for you, so be sure to check all the chapters.

Look at the photos of referral patterns in each chapter, and try to find the ones that most closely match your pain pattern. Read the list of symptoms for each muscle. Do any of the referral patterns look familiar? Do any of the symptoms sound familiar? These are the ones you want to work on first.

Be sure to go back and read all of the chapters, because those trigger points may also play a role in your pain. You may need to work on all the listed muscles if you are not sure which muscle contains the trigger points that are causing your pain, or because trigger points in more than one muscle may be causing your pain.

You may wish to make copies of the blank body chart on page 78 and draw your symptom pattern on it with a colored marker. Then you can compare it with the pain referral pictures in chapters 9 through 23. Out to the side of each painful area, note your pain intensity on a scale of 1 to 10 and the percent of time you feel pain in that area, for example, "6.5/80%."

I recommend that you fill out a body chart at least a couple of times per week. Date them so you'll be able to keep them in order. This chronological record will come in handy in several ways: It will make it easier to discern which patterns fit your pain referral most closely. It will also help you recognize the factors that cause and perpetuate your symptoms by matching fluctuations in the level and frequency of your symptoms. And finally, it will allow you to track your progress (or lack thereof) and provide a historical record of any injuries. As your condition improves, you may forget how intense your symptoms were originally, and you may think you're not getting any

The muscle names are followed by the chapter number

1. Quadriceps Femoris Muscles (10)
   Adductors Longus & Brevis (11)

2. Vastus Lateralis (10)

3. Gastrocnemius (15)
   Hamstring Muscles (13)
   Popliteus (14)
   Soleus (16)

4. Quadriceps Femoris Muscles (10)
   Adductor Muscles of the Hip (11)
   Sartorius (12)

5. Tibialis Anterior (19)
   Adductors Longus & Brevis (11)

6. Gastrocnemius (15)
   Gluteus Minimus (9)
   Peroneus Longus & Brevis (18)
   Vastus Lateralis (10)

7. Soleus (16)
   Gastrocnemius (15)
   Gluteus Minimus (9)
   Semimembranosus
   & Semitendinosus (13)
   Flexor Digitorum Longus (20)
   Tibialis Posterior (17)

8. Tibialis Anterior (19)
   Peroneus Tertius (18)
   Long Extensor Muscles
   of the Toes (21)

9. Peroneal Muscles (18)

10. Soleus (16)
    Tibialis Posterior (17)

11. Abductor Hallucis (22)
    Flexor Digitorum
    Longus (20)

12. Extensors Digitorum Brevis
    and Hallucis Brevis (22)
    Long Extensor
    Muscles of the Toes (21)
    Deep Intrinsic
    Foot Muscles (23)
    Tibialis Anterior (19)

13. Tibialis Anterior (19)
    Extensor Hallucis
    Longus (21)
    Flexor Hallucis Brevis (23)

14. Foot Interossei (23)
    Extensor Digitorum
    Longus (21)

15. Soleus (16)
    Quadratus Plantae (23)
    Abductor Hallucis (22)
    Tibialis Posterior (17)

16. Gastrocnemius (15)
    Flexor Digitorum
    Longus (20)
    Deep Intrinsic
    Foot Muscles (23)
    Soleus (16)
    Abductor Hallucis (22)
    Tibialis Posterior (17)

17. Deep Intrinsic Foot
    Muscles (23)
    Superficial Intrinsic Foot
    Muscles (22)
    Long Flexor Muscles
    of the Toes (20)
    Tibialis Posterior (17)

18. Flexor Hallucis Longus (20)
    Flexor Hallucis Brevis (23)
    Tibialis Posterior (17)

19. Flexor Digitorum
    Longus (20)
    Tibialis Posterior (17)

better. The body charts will help prevent this frustration by graphically illustrating any reduction in the overall intensity or frequency of your pain and the extent of the area affected. You'll be able to see that you are improving, even if you have an occasional setback. One note: not everyone can accurately draw their pain location, due in part to lack of familiarity with anatomy, so take that possibility into consideration and check muscles with adjacent referral patterns just in case your drawing is inaccurate.

Muscle Chapters

Chapters 9 through 23 cover the major muscles commonly associated with lower leg, knee, ankle, or foot pain and other symptoms. Each chapter contains an anatomical drawing of the muscle or muscles covered in that chapter. Photographs show the most common pain referral areas for each trigger point. The more solid black overlay area indicates the primary area of referral, which is almost always present, and the stippled area shows the most likely secondary areas of referral, which may or may not be present. The letter X marks spots where trigger points are most commonly found in conjunction with that referral pattern. There may be additional trigger points, so search the entire muscle.

The pain referral photographs in the muscle chapters show only the most common referral patterns; bear in mind that your referral pattern may be somewhat different or even completely different. Also, you may have overlapping referral patterns from trigger points in multiple muscles. These areas may be larger than the patterns common for individual muscles, so be sure to search for trigger points in all the muscles that refer pain to that area. Pain may be particularly intense in areas where you have overlapping pain referral.

In the following chapters, the information for each muscle includes lists of common symptoms and causes or perpetuators of trigger points. Again, these are only the most common; you may experience different symptoms, and your causes and perpetuating factors may be different. If you suspect trigger points in a certain muscle but don't see any causes listed that seem to apply to you, try to imagine whether anything in your life is similar to something on the list, in effect causing the same type of stress on the muscle. For example, perhaps you don't wear high heels, but you might be an ice skater, which requires side-to-side balance over a thin blade. This would stress the peroneal muscles on the outside of the lower leg.

Each muscle chapter provides stretches for the muscle or muscles covered in that chapter. If you're seeing a practitioner, have them check to make sure you're performing the stretches properly. If your symptoms are getting worse, stop doing the self-help techniques and consult with your practitioner.

Conclusion

Once you've determined which two muscles most closely fit your pain pattern, start working on those. Over the next several weeks, start treating additional muscles. Periodically review the guidelines in chapter 7 to make sure you're doing the self-treatments properly. As you start to feel better, you'll develop a clearer picture of which trigger points in which muscles are causing your pain, and which perpetuating factors are reactivating your trigger points.

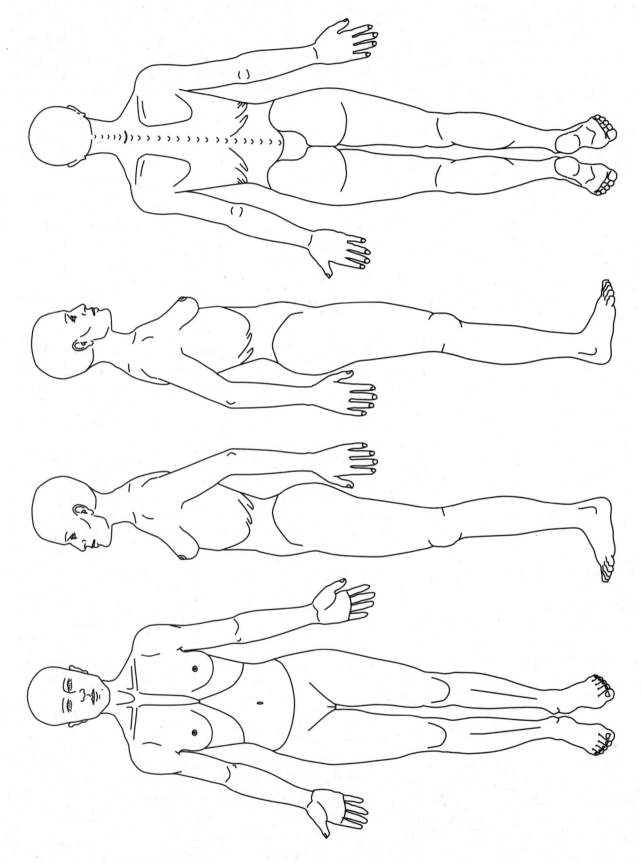

Chapter 9

Gluteus Minimus

Referred pain from trigger points in the gluteus minimus muscle is frequently diagnosed by both patients and health care practitioners as "sciatic pain" because of the distribution pattern down the side and back of the leg. One study showed that at least 79 percent of pain down the leg comes from trigger point referral from either the gluteus minimus or piriformis muscles, and not from "pinched nerves," a herniated disk, or stenosis in a lumbar vertebra. (Stenosis is a narrowing of either the big hole in the vertebra that the spinal cord goes through, or a narrowing of the smaller holes the nerves travel through.) Since sciatica is usually assumed to be caused by compression of a nerve, referred pain from trigger points is probably more aptly called "pseudosciatica."

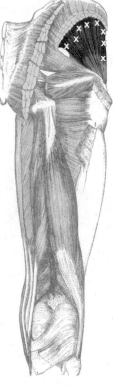

If your pain truly comes from compression of a lumbar nerve, you would probably draw your referral pattern as a thin line that starts from a very specific spot on one side of a lumbar vertebra, and then continues into the gluteal area and down the leg. That pain is usually sharper and more intense than this type. If your pain referral starts in the gluteal area and not a pinpoint spot in the lumbar area, it is likely caused by trigger points.

Common Symptoms

- Trigger points in the anterior portion of the muscle (on your side, under the seam of your pants) refer pain down the side of your leg to your ankle, and possibly to a spot on the backside of your buttocks.

- Trigger points in the posterior portion of the muscle (partway between your side and your backside) refer pain over the gluteal area and down the back of your leg into your calf.

- Pain in your hip may cause you to walk with a limp.

- Sleeping on the same side as the trigger points may cause pain severe enough to wake you.

- You may have difficulty rising out of a chair after sitting for a while.

- You may have difficulty in finding a comfortable position standing, walking, or lying down.

- You probably experience pain while running or hiking.

Possible Causes and Perpetuators

Postural

- Sitting with a wallet in your back pocket

- Walking with a limp from an injury

- Sitting for too long, especially when driving

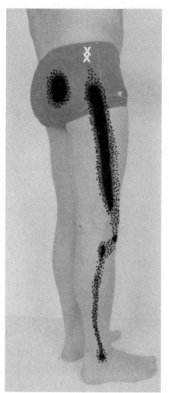

Gluteus minimus—
anterior portion

Injuries or Muscle Abuse

- Suddenly overexerting your muscle when it's not used to it, such as when taking up a new sport

- Overusing the muscle chronically while playing tennis, racquetball, or handball, or while walking or running too far or too fast too often, especially on rough ground

- Standing for long periods with your weight shifted to one side or with your feet too close together

- Falling and landing on your gluteal area or your back, or a near-fall that causes you to use the muscle suddenly

Medical or Structural

- Having a sacroiliac joint (the joint where the sacrum and big pelvic bone join) that is out of alignment

- Irritation of a nerve root

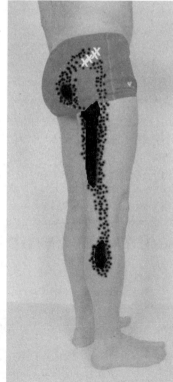

Gluteus minimus—
posterior portion

- Injections of medications, especially irritants, which can cause pain that lasts for months

- Overloading your muscles due to obesity

- Chilling of your gluteus minimus muscle or your body as a whole

- Having a small hemipelvis (the left or right portion of the pelvis; see page 40)

Helpful Hints

Don't carry a wallet in your back pocket, since this tilts your pelvis and leads to problems in muscles throughout your body.

If you must stand for long periods, stand with your feet apart and shift your weight frequently from one foot to the other. If you sit for long periods, move around the room every fifteen to twenty minutes. A timer set across the room ensures that you will get up periodically to turn it off.

Sleep with a pillow between your legs until your pain is resolved, as this will help take pressure off the muscle.

Runners and avid hikers usually have gluteus minimus trigger points. Back off on your runs or hikes until the trigger points have improved dramatically. You can then *slowly* increase your mileage, staying out of the pain zone. I recommend doing both the ball self-work and ample stretching before and after your run. If you are obese, don't overdo exercising these muscles until trigger points have been inactivated and strength is built up gradually. Walk with a wider stance.

Keep these muscles warm; if possible, keep your entire body warm.

See a chiropractor or osteopathic physician to check your sacroiliac joint and lumbar vertebrae for alignment problems. If you have a small hemipelvis or some other structural imbalance, see a specialist for compensating lifts and pads. If you have had a laminectomy surgery and still have remaining pain, check the gluteus minimus for trigger points.

If you receive muscular injections, avoid this muscle. Inject into the gluteus medius and deltoid muscles, since they are less prone to developing trigger points.

Self-Help Techniques

Applying Pressure

Gluteus Minimus Pressure

Common trigger points in the gluteus minimus are found in the upper third of the backside of your gluteal area, to over on your side between your hip joint and the top of your pelvis. Lying face up, lie on a tennis ball and move it with your hand while searching for trigger points.

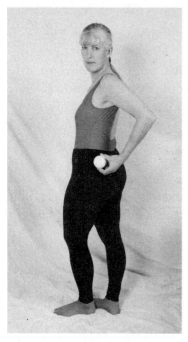

Area to work for gluteus minimus—posterior portion

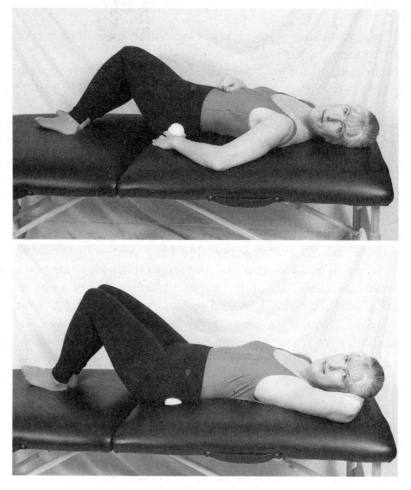

Start moving out onto your side. By the time you work on the entire muscle, you will be lying on your side. Many patients make the mistake of not getting far enough forward. If you end up working over the seam of your pants, you are getting all the points; otherwise, keep searching farther forward. Be sure to work on the gluteus minimus muscles on *both* the right and left sides of your body.

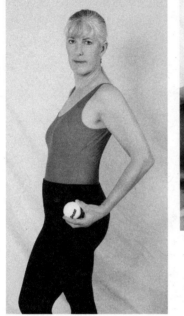

Area to work for gluteus minimus—anterior portion

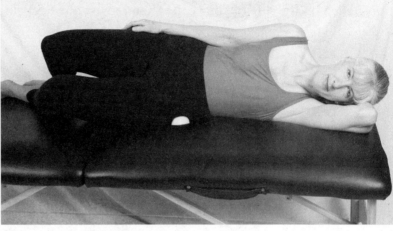

Stretches

Gluteus Minimus Stretch, Anterior Muscle Portion

To stretch the *anterior* fibers of the gluteus minimus muscle, lie on your side on the edge of your bed with your back scooted right up to the edge. Allow your top leg to drop behind you, off the edge. Allow gravity to give you a stretch. If you want more of a stretch, put the heel of your opposite leg on the side of your calf. Then move your heel closer to your knee for an even greater stretch.

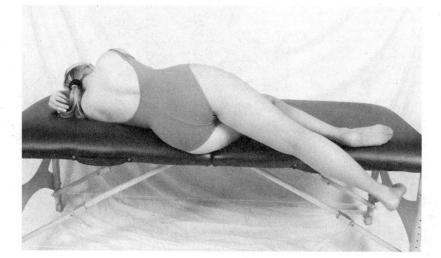

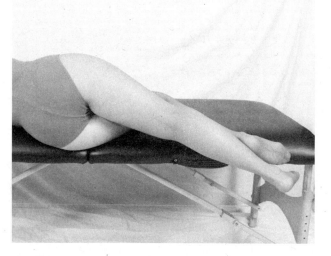
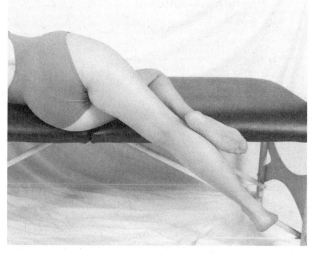

Gluteus Minimus Stretch, Posterior Muscle Portion

To stretch the *posterior* fibers of the gluteus minimus muscle, lie on your side and position yourself on the end of the bed with the leg/hip being stretched out over the end of the bed and slightly forward of the line of your trunk, with your toes slightly rotated toward the floor. Your bottom leg is bent at more than 90 degrees (so that it is still mostly on the bed). Let gravity give you a stretch.

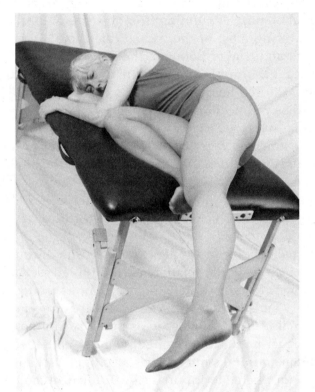

Also See

- Quadriceps Muscles: see vastus lateralis; satellite trigger points can develop here

- Peroneal Muscles: see peroneus longus

Conclusion

Trigger points in the piriformis muscle can cause a referral pattern similar to gluteus minimus trigger points, but the most common referred pain tends to run down the back of the thigh instead of out toward the side. Trigger points in the quadratus lumborum muscles (in the lumbar area) may keep gluteus minimus muscle trigger points active, so it is worth considering that there may be trigger points in these muscles that need to be relieved. Tightness in the opposite thorocolumbar paraspinal muscles (a set of muscles running from the base of the skull to the top of the pelvis and from the spine out, covering most of the back of the thorax) can tilt and rotate the pelvis, causing pain in the hip joint and trigger points in the gluteal muscles. Since these trigger points don't directly cause lower leg, knee, ankle, or foot pain, they are not addressed in this book. If you can't relieve your pain with the self-help techniques in this book within six to eight weeks, you may wish to consider whether you need to treat trigger points in the piriformis, quadratus lumborum, and/or paraspinal muscles. See the Resources section for books and other resources that provide guidance on self-treatment of muscles not covered in this book.

If your pain does start next to a lumbar vertebra and not in the gluteal area, you need to see a doctor and get an MRI to be evaluated for disk problems and stenosis. Acupuncture will help heal disk problems, but stenosis may require surgery. These surgeries have become very sophisticated in the last few years and often have you back on your feet within a day or two, depending on the area of the stenosis.

If the pain is very localized over the hip joint or perhaps from the buttocks down the side to the trochanteric knee, it may be bursitis (inflammation of a fluid-filled sac over the bony prominence of the femur called the trochanter that allows the gluteus minimus tendon to glide over the trochanter). The hip joint will be very tender to pressure, and pressure reproduces the symptoms. Gluteus minimus trigger points can also be misdiagnosed as bursitis, so it is always worth checking the surrounding muscles for trigger points and seeing if you can get relief. In every case of *true* bursitis I have treated, the gluteus minimus muscle was also tight, so I suspect tightness and trigger points are a causative factor for trochanteric bursitis. Acupuncture can help treat the inflammation of true bursitis along with treating the trigger points in the surrounding muscles.

Chapter 10

Quadriceps Femoris Muscle Group

The quadriceps femoris muscle group includes the rectus femoris, vastus medialis, vastus intermedius, and the vastus lateralis. Trigger points in the quadriceps femoris muscles are very common and are frequently overlooked, mainly because they only minimally restrict range of motion, if at all. If you have weakness when extending your knee, you probably have either active or latent trigger points in the rectus femoris, vastus medialis, and/or vastus intermedius.

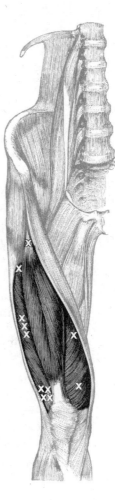

Common Symptoms

Rectus Femoris

- Trigger points cause pain deep in your knee, in and around your kneecap, and possibly on the front of your thigh at night in bed. Even though the pain is primarily in the knee area, the trigger point is just below the crease of the groin.

- Occasionally you may find a trigger point just above the knee, which will refer pain deep into the knee joint.

- Going down stairs is more likely to be a problem than going up stairs.

- In above-knee amputees, phantom limb pain may come from trigger points in the rectus femoris, particularly if the muscle was stretched to cover the bone.

Vastus Medialis

- The trigger point closer to the knee refers pain to the front of your knee, and the trigger point about midthigh refers pain over the inside of your knee and thigh.

- Toothache-like pain deep in the knee joint can interrupt your sleep, and may be misdiagnosed as inflammation of the knee.

- Trigger points only minimally restrict range of motion and may only affect your leg function rather than causing pain.

- You may experience unexpected "buckling of the knee" (usually when walking on rough ground) produced by muscle weakness, which can lead to falls and injury.

- If trigger points are present in both the vastus medialis and the rectus femoris, your hip may buckle unexpectedly.

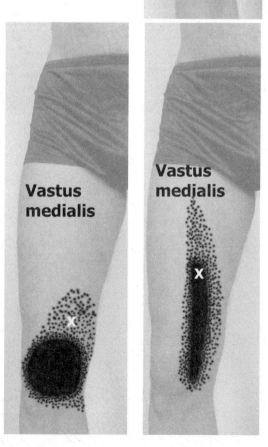

Rectus femoris

Vastus medialis

Vastus medialis

Vastus Intermedius

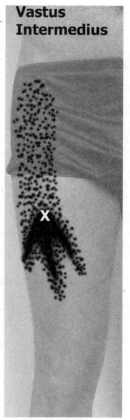

Vastus Intermedius

- Trigger points cause intense pain at your midthigh, closer to the outside of the thigh.

- Pain usually occurs with movement, and rarely with rest.

- You may have difficulty fully straightening your knee, which causes you to limp when walking, especially after sitting for a while.

- You may have difficulty with climbing stairs.

- A "buckling knee" can be caused by a combination of trigger points in the vastus intermedius and the two heads of the gastrocnemius below the crease on the back side of your knee.

- Trigger points can cause your kneecap to lock, though this is more commonly caused by trigger points in the vastus lateralis muscle.

- Vastus intermedius trigger points develop secondary to trigger points in the other muscles of the quadriceps femoris group.

Vastus Lateralis

- The vastus lateralis develops multiple trigger points along the outside of your thigh, causing a variety of referral patterns along the outside of your thigh, knee, and possibly down into your calf.

- You probably experience pain with walking, and you may drag your foot on the affected side.

- Pain may disturb your sleep when you are lying on the involved side.

- A "stuck patella" (kneecap) can cause difficulty in straightening or bending your knee after getting up from a chair.

- If your kneecap is completely locked, your knee will be slightly bent and you will not be able to walk or sit without your leg supported in the locked position.

- Going up stairs is more likely to be a problem than going down stairs.

- Trigger point referral can be misdiagnosed as trochanteric bursitis if pain is referred over the outside of the hip bone (the greater trochanter).

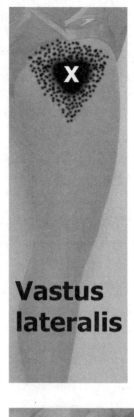

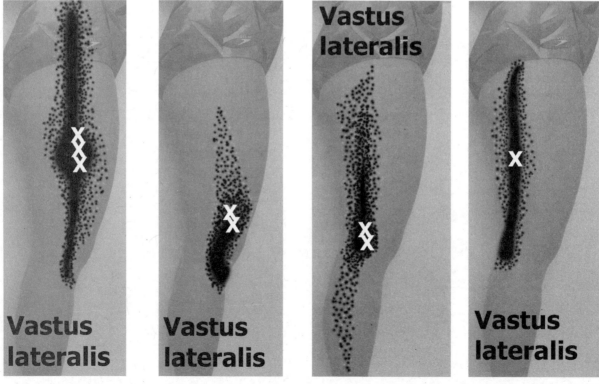

Ligamentous Trigger Point

- The lateral collateral ligament may refer pain to an area just above it on the outside of your knee.

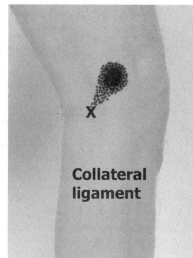

Collateral ligament

Possible Causes and Perpetuators

Postural

- Sitting with one foot under your buttocks

- Sitting for a long time with a heavy weight on your lap (rectus femoris)

- Kneeling on a hard surface (vastus medialis)

- Sitting for a long period with your leg out straight (vastus lateralis)

Injuries or Muscle Abuse

- Stumbling, such as into a hole or off a curb

- Doing strenuous athletic activities such as jogging, skiing, football, basketball, and soccer (vastus medialis)

- Suddenly overloading the muscles during sports, causing injuries

- Receiving a direct blow to the front or sides of your thigh, or your knee joint

- Doing deep knee bends

- Doing knee extensions with a weight near your ankle (see a physical therapist for a proper way to do this exercise)

- Falling (vastus medialis)

- Fracturing a hip and/or having hip surgery (rectus femoris)

- Wearing a cast on your leg, or any other lengthy immobilization

- Tightness in the hamstring muscles

- Active trigger points in the soleus muscle, which restrict the motion of the ankle and lead to overload of the quadriceps femoris group

- Injecting drugs, such as insulin, into the thigh

Medical or Structural

- Degenerative hip joint disease (rectus femoris and vastus lateralis)

- Abnormal hip joint mechanics (rectus femoris and vastus lateralis)

- Excessive foot pronation (vastus medialis)

- Flat feet, which leads to pronation (vastus medialis)

Helpful Hints

Don't wear high heels.

Don't kneel for long periods. Sit on a low stool instead, and take frequent breaks. Do not do deep knee bends or squats, and avoid picking things up off the floor.

Avoid sitting in the same position for extended periods, especially with your thighs at less than a 90-degree angle to your trunk. Be sure to use a lumbar support.

Don't sit with your legs extended straight out in front of you, or with your foot under your buttocks. Sitting in a rocking chair helps keep your muscles mobilized. When getting out of a chair, use your arms to assist you in rising. When driving, use a lumbar support and something like a pillow under your buttocks to increase the angle between your torso and thighs. Take frequent breaks.

If you have trigger points in the vastus medialis or vastus lateralis, sleep on the unaffected side with a pillow between your legs. Don't bring your thighs up toward your chest, and don't straighten your legs out all the way either.

Warm up properly for athletic activities. In the initial stages of treatment, you may wish to wear a neoprene knee brace, which will help remind you to be careful with your leg and will maintain warmth around the lower ends of these muscles.

It is important to identify and treat any lumbar vertebrae that are out of alignment and any hip alignment problems. See a chiropractor or osteopathic physician for evaluation and treatment.

Get corrective orthotics to solve foot pronation problems. If one leg is shorter than the other, see a specialist to get a compensating lift.

Self-Help Techniques

Caution: Do not apply pressure to your legs if you have varicose veins in the area to be treated— it could release a clot that could go to your heart or brain! *An acupuncturist or massage therapist should treat your legs, because they can avoid the veins.* You may still do the stretches below.

Treat the hamstrings first (chapter 13) to avoid the cramping that can be caused by releasing the quadriceps femoris group. If you don't find trigger points in the hamstrings, you can probably skip this step in the future.

Applying Pressure

Vastus Lateralis Pressure

To work on the vastus lateralis, start with the gluteus minimus (anterior portion) self-help ball work (chapter 9). Then continue on down the side of your thigh, using your hand to move the tennis ball as you search for tender points. Be sure to work the whole length of the muscle.

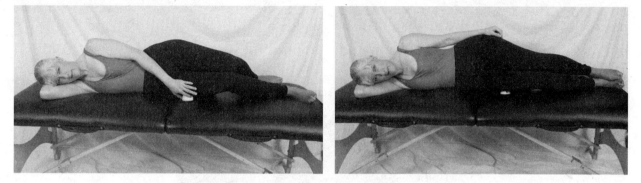

There may be some trigger points under the edge of the kneecap. Straighten out your leg most of the way, wrap your hands around your knee, and put both thumbs on the edge of the kneecap. Press the kneecap away from you while simultaneously pressing into trigger points in that area.

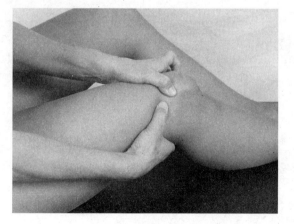

Rectus Femoris and Vastus Intermedius Pressure

To work on the rectus femoris and the underlying vastus intermedius, roll onto your stomach and, with your leg bent, move the tennis ball around, checking for tender points. Be sure to work the entire length of the muscle.

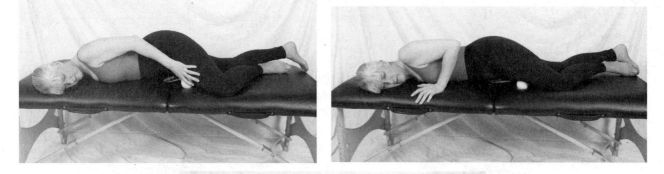

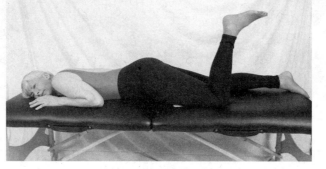

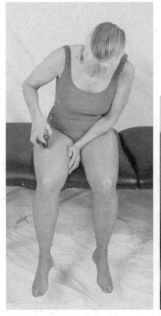

As an alternative, hold a golf ball or other pressure device in the center of your palm and press into tender points. This is less effective than lying on the ball due to the thickness of the rectus femoris.

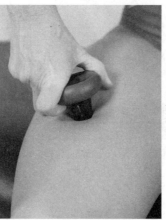

Vastus Medialis Pressure

To work on the vastus medialis, hold a golf ball or other pressure device in the center of the palm of your opposite hand to press into tender points. You may also use your opposite thumb. It does not take a lot of pressure to treat these trigger points.

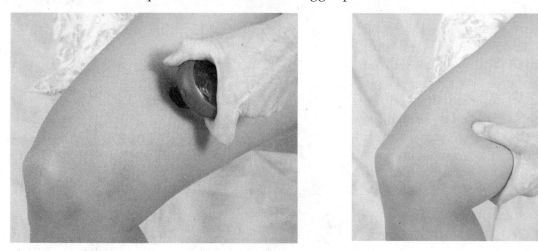

Stretches

Quadriceps Side-Lying Stretch

Lying in bed on your side, bend the bottom leg to almost a 90-degree angle to the trunk so you can rest your top leg on the bottom leg. Grab the ankle of the upper leg and pull it up behind you so you are getting a stretch on the front of the thigh. Turn over and stretch the other thigh.

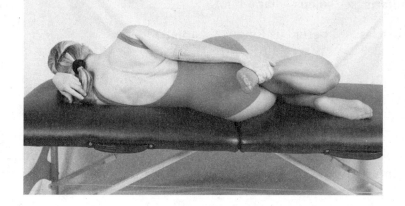

Quadriceps Standing Stretch

When standing, grab the ankle using the hand on the same side, and pull the leg up behind you. Be sure to hold onto a counter or a nonmobile piece of furniture for support. Then with the same hand, grab the opposite ankle and pull the leg up behind you. Repeat on the other side. The first part emphasizes the stretch of the vastus medialis, and the second part emphasizes the stretch of the vastus lateralis. This stretch is most effective when done in a warm swimming pool, holding onto the edge for balance.

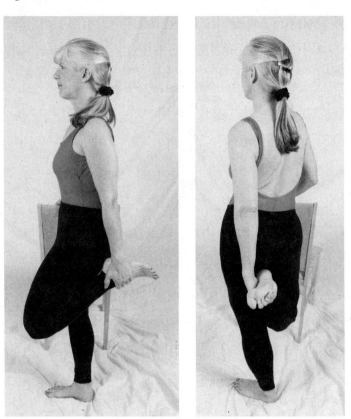

Also See

- Hamstrings (chapter 13)

- Sartorius (chapter 12)

- Gluteus Minimus: see anterior portion (chapter 9)

- Adductor Muscles of the Hip (chapter 11)

- Soleus/Plantaris: see soleus (chapter 16)

- Peroneal Muscles: see peroneus longus (chapter 18)

Conclusion

You may need to search for trigger points in the gluteus minimus muscle (anterior portion), since they can cause a referral pattern similar to vastus lateralis trigger points and may also keep vastus lateralis trigger points activated. If you feel pain on the front or inside of your thigh, also search the adductor muscles of the hip (adductors longus and/or brevis and gracilis). You will also need to search the hamstrings and soleus muscles, since they can activate and perpetuate trigger points in the quadriceps femoris group. If you find trigger points in the rectus femoris muscle, also search the others in the quadriceps group as well as the sartorius. If you find trigger points in the vastus medialis, also search the rectus femoris (this chapter), peroneus longus, and adductor muscles of the hip. If you find trigger points in the vastus intermedius, also search the rectus femoris and vastus lateralis.

Trigger points in the tensor fasciae latae (upper thigh, toward the outside) and iliopsoas muscles (deep in the abdominal and pelvic areas) can also refer into the thigh in some of the same areas as the quadriceps femoris muscles, but since these trigger points don't directly cause lower leg, knee, ankle, or foot pain, they are not addressed in this book. If you can't relieve your pain with the self-help techniques in this book within six to eight weeks, you may wish to consider whether you need to treat trigger points in these other muscles. See the Resources section for books and other resources that can provide guidance on self-treatment of muscles not covered in this book.

A buckling knee can also be caused by anterior subluxation of the lateral tibial plateau (deep in the knee joint), which requires surgical correction. But since trigger points in the vastus medialis are the more likely culprits, search that muscle first. Trigger points in the upper part of the vastus lateralis commonly get misdiagnosed as trochanteric bursitis. See the gluteus minimus muscle (chapter 9) for more information on bursitis.

As you may recall from chapter 3, there are many causes of knee pain, including ligament strains and tears, torn menisci, osteoarthritis, tendinopathies, bursitis, and kneecap fractures. If you still have pain after inactivating trigger points, you will need to see an orthopedic doctor for evaluation. Even if other causes are found, there are also likely trigger points involved, and treatment can help prepare you both for surgery and for recovery afterward.

Chapter 11

Adductor Muscles of the Hip

The adductor muscles of the hip include the adductor longus, adductor brevis, adductor magnus, and gracilis. These muscles allow you to bring your leg toward the opposite leg.

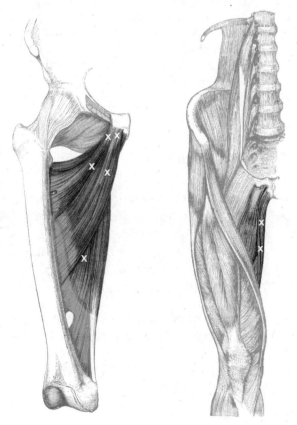

Common Symptoms

Adductor Longus and Adductor Brevis

- Trigger points refer pain on the front of your thigh, over the front of your knee, and down the inside of your lower leg, and the pain feels deep.

- Trigger points may cause knee stiffness.

- You may feel pain only during vigorous activity or when overloading the muscle.

- Pain is increased by standing and by sudden twists of your hip.

- You may experience restricted range of motion when moving your thigh away from the midline of your body.

- You may experience restricted range of motion when rotating your thigh outward.

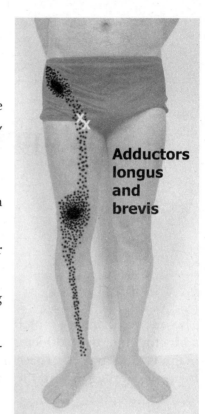

Adductors longus and brevis

Adductor Magnus

- Trigger points refer pain on the front-inside of the thigh, from the groin area down to the inside of your knee, and the pain feels deep, possibly like it's shooting up into your pelvis and exploding like a firecracker.

- A trigger point high up between the legs, where the muscle attaches to the "sit bone" (ischial tuberosity), may refer pain to the pubic bone, vagina, rectum, or possibly the bladder.

- Pain may occur only during intercourse.

- You may have difficulty getting comfortable at night.

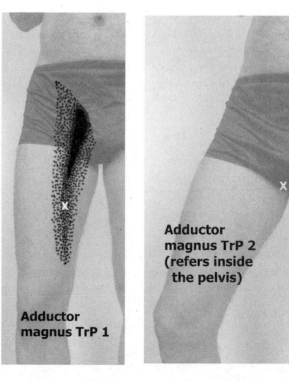

Adductor magnus TrP 1

Adductor magnus TrP 2 (refers inside the pelvis)

Gracilis

- Trigger points refer pain on the inside of your thigh that feels hot, stinging, and superficial.

- Pain may be constant at rest, and no change of position relieves it except for walking.

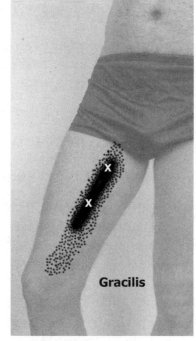

Gracilis

Possible Causes and Perpetuators

Postural

- Sitting for long periods, especially when driving, or with one leg crossed over your other knee.

Injuries or Muscle Abuse

- A sudden overload, for example, trying to stop yourself from slipping on ice by trying to keep your legs from spreading

- Horseback riding

- Riding on long bike trips, if you haven't trained for it

- Running up or down hills

- Skiing, most likely by snowplowing/wedge turns, or unexpectedly doing the "splits"

Helpful Hints

When sleeping, put a pillow between your knees, and try to keep your upper leg almost straight. Don't sit with your legs crossed, and if you must sit for long periods, stand and move around frequently.

Apply moist heat to your upper front and inner thigh.

Be sure to reread part II on perpetuating factors, particularly the sections on infections, nutritional problems, and organ dysfunction and disease.

Self-Help Techniques

Caution: Do not apply pressure to your legs if you have varicose veins in the area to be treated—it could release a clot that could go to your heart or brain! *An acupuncturist or massage therapist should treat your legs, because they can avoid the veins.* You may still do the stretches below.

Applying Pressure

Adductor Muscles of the Hip Pressure

Sit with your legs bent to one side, with one heel close to the pubic area and the other one

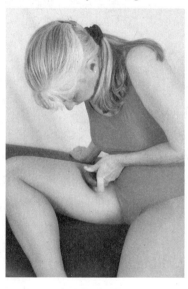 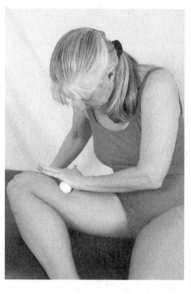

out to the side. Using a golf ball or other pressure device in the center of your palm, press the device into tender points on your inner thigh.

To access the upper portion of the adductor magnus, reach between your legs, and find your "sit bone" with your fingers. Press the muscle attachment all around that area. It is easiest to use the hand of the opposite side. In addition to applying pressure to the adductor muscles, you may be able to lift and pinch part of this muscle group between your thumb and fingers, using your opposite hand.

Stretches

Rotating Adductor Stretch

Hold onto a chair back, spread your legs apart almost as far as you can with your toes pointed forward, and gently rotate your pelvis away from the side you are stretching.

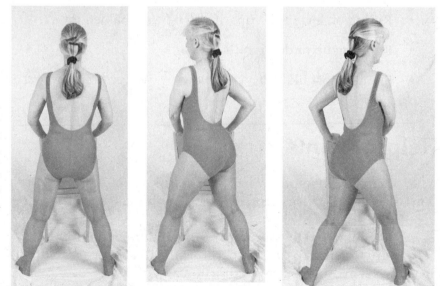

Adductor Stretch to Side

Hold onto a chair back, spread your legs apart almost as far as you can, and shift your weight to one side, allowing that knee to bend. You should feel a stretch on the opposite inner thigh. This stretch can also be done in a warm swimming pool in chest-deep water, which may be easier on your knees.

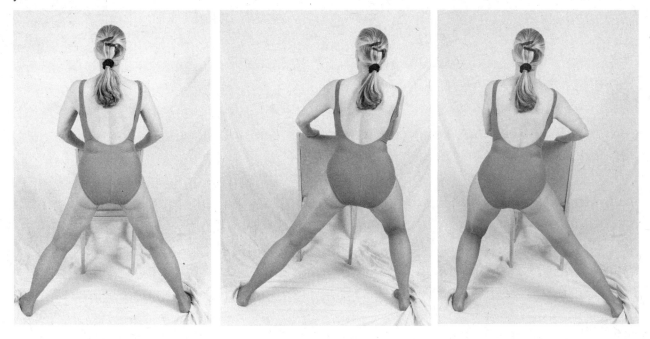

Also See

- Quadriceps Femoris: see vastus lateralis (chapter 10)

Conclusion

The portions of the adductor muscles of the hip that are close to the pubic bone are more difficult to treat on yourself, so you will probably also need the help of a massage therapist, acupuncturist, or physical therapist to treat all of the trigger points. Since the adductor magnus muscle is so deep, it is hard to work on with self-help techniques only. Ultrasound is an effective treatment.

If you get pain in the low back / upper gluteal area after working on the hip adductors, you may need to search for trigger points in the gluteus medius muscle. You may need to work on this muscle first in the future. Since trigger points in the gluteus medius muscle don't directly cause lower leg, knee, ankle, or foot pain, they are not addressed in this book. If you can't relieve your pain with the self-help techniques in this book within six to eight weeks, you may wish to consider whether you need to treat trigger points in this muscle. See the Resources section for books and other resources that can provide guidance on self-treatment of muscles not covered in this book.

Chapter 12

Sartorius

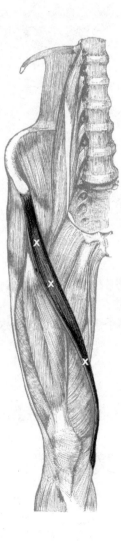

Common Symptoms

- Trigger points refer pain that is superficial, sharp, and tingling, and felt at various points in the front of your thigh, and may also cause superficial pain on the inside of your knee.

- If the lateral femoral cutaneous nerve is entrapped, you may feel numbness, burning, or uncomfortable sensations in the front of your thigh (meralgia paresthetica), which will be increased by standing or walking.

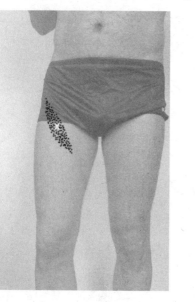 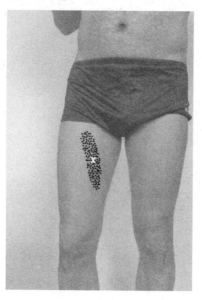 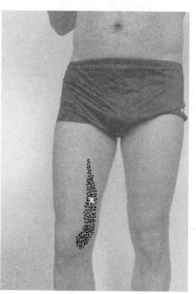

Possible Causes and Perpetuators

Injuries or Muscle Abuse

- A twisting fall

Medical or Structural

- Excessive foot pronation

Other

- Trigger points are usually found in conjunction with trigger points in other muscles (see below).

Helpful Hints

Don't sit cross-legged in the lotus position, or with your ankle crossed over your opposite knee. Don't sleep with your knees drawn up tightly toward your chest. Place a pillow between your legs.

If you have burning pain or odd sensations on the front of your thigh, try searching for trigger points below the pointy bony part of the front of your pelvis. Meralgia paresthetica (see above in "Common Symptoms") may be caused by obesity, constricting garments or belts, one leg being anatomically shorter than the other, or carrying a wallet in your front pants pocket. These causes will need to be addressed in order to obtain lasting relief.

Self-Help Techniques

Applying Pressure

Sartorius Pressure

You may use the same pressure techniques as for the vastus medialis and rectus femoris muscles (chapter 10), and you may also massage the muscle. Note how the muscle goes from the pointy part of the hip bone in front, crosses the front of the thigh, and then curves into your inner thigh as it approaches the knee. Be sure to work on all those areas so you won't miss any part of the muscle.

Also See

- Quadriceps Femoris: see rectus femoris and vastus medialis (chapter 10)

- Adductor Muscles of the Hip (chapter 11)

Conclusion

Trigger points in the lower part of the sartorius muscle refer pain in an area similar to the vastus medialis, but pain from vastus medialis trigger points will feel deeper in the knee joint rather than diffuse and superficial.

The sartorius muscle rarely develops trigger points on its own. Usually there are also trigger points in the quadriceps femoris muscles (rectus femoris and vastus medialis), iliopsoas, pectineus, tensor fasciae latae, and/or adductor muscles of the hip. Since trigger points in the iliopsoas, pectineus (a short muscle running from the lower pelvis to the top of the femur), and tensor fasciae latae don't directly cause lower leg, knee, ankle, or foot pain, they are not addressed in this book. If you can't relieve your pain with the self-help techniques in this book within six to eight weeks, you may wish to consider whether you need to treat trigger points in these other muscles. See the Resources section for books and other resources that can provide guidance on self-treatment of muscles not covered in this book.

<h1 style="text-align:center">Chapter 13</h1>

<h1 style="text-align:center">Hamstrings Muscle Group</h1>

The hamstrings muscle group includes the biceps femoris, semitendinosus, and semimembranosus.

Referred pain from trigger points in the hamstring muscles frequently is diagnosed by both patients and practitioners as "sciatic pain," because of the distribution pattern down the back of the leg. One study (Travell and Simons 1992) showed that 79 percent of pain down the leg comes from trigger point referral, not from "pinched nerves," a herniated disk, or stenosis in a lumbar vertebra, though from my experience this number may be even higher. Since sciatica is usually assumed to be caused by compression on a nerve, pain referral from trigger points is probably more aptly called "pseudosciatica."

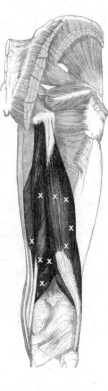

Common Symptoms

- Trigger points refer pain over the back of your thigh, around the crease of your butt, over the back of your knee, and sometimes over your calf.

- You may have pain with walking, possibly even causing a limp, and pain with getting up from a chair, particularly if your legs have been crossed.

- You will probably feel pain on the back of your thigh, in your knee, and in the crease area of your butt when sitting, due to pressure on the trigger points. You may experience tingling and numbness when sitting in a chair that is too high.

- You may have restricted range of motion when attempting to bend forward to reach your toes.

- Pain in the biceps femoris muscle can disrupt your sleep.

- It may feel like the pain is *only* in the quadriceps femoris muscle on the front of your thigh (chapter 10), when in fact the problem originates in the hamstrings and causes trigger points to form in the quadriceps femoris group.

- In above-knee amputees, phantom limb pain may come from trigger points in the hamstrings, particularly if the muscle was stretched to cover the bone.

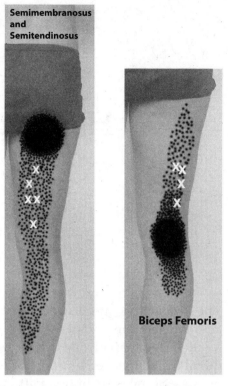

Possible Causes and Perpetuators

Postural

- Sitting in a chair where your feet don't touch the ground, which is more common in shorter people.

- For children, sitting in a high chair without a footrest

- Sitting on a ski lift without a footrest

Injuries or Muscle Abuse

- Inadequate stretching before a sports activity, resulting in a strain or partial tear of the hamstrings

- Treating quadriceps femoris trigger points without also treating the hamstrings

- Auto accidents, regardless of the direction of impact

Medical or Structural

- Having a small hemipelvis (see page 40)

- Having short upper arms in relation to torso height, causing you to shift your weight forward when sitting

Helpful Hints

If your chair is too high for you (you should be able to easily slip your fingers between your chair and thigh), buy or build a sloped footstool. Patio chairs can cause problems if there is a metal bar across the front of the chair (behind your knees) and a sagging seat bottom. When driving for long periods, use cruise control and take frequent breaks.

Make sure children in high chairs have footrests and those at school have chairs or footrests of the proper height.

If you swim, don't use the crawl stroke too much, but instead alternate it with other strokes. If you bicycle, be sure your seat height is set high enough that your legs can straighten out as much as possible without your knees locking.

If you have pain remaining after a laminectomy, check the hamstrings for trigger points.

Self-Help Techniques

Caution: Do not apply pressure to your legs if you have varicose veins in the area to be treated— it could release a clot that could go to your heart or brain! *An acupuncturist or massage therapist should treat your legs, because they can avoid the veins.* You may still do the stretch below.

Applying Pressure

Hamstrings Muscles Pressure

Sit on a surface where your legs can dangle but are fully supported the length of the thigh. Place a tennis ball under one thigh, and use your hand to move the ball around to tender points. Repeat on the opposite thigh.

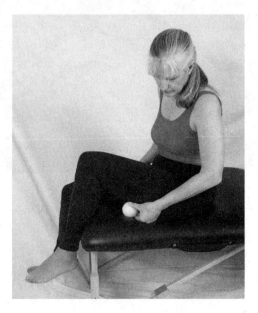
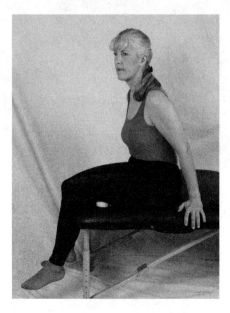

You may also treat the inner-thigh hamstrings by using your opposite hand to pinch the muscles between your thumb and fingers.

Stretches

Hamstrings/Calves Stretch

Sit with your legs out straight in front of you. With your head hanging forward as far as is comfortable, lean forward and reach your hands down toward your toes, until you get a gentle stretch. Relax and then repeat, moving your hands farther down each time, but only as far down as you can get a gentle stretch. Do this in a hot bath if you can.

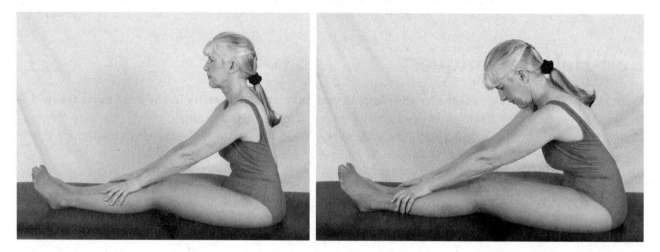

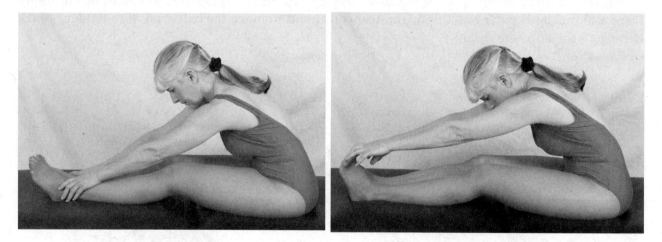

Also See

- Gluteus Minimus: see posterior portion (chapter 9)

- Quadriceps Femoris: see vastus lateralis (chapter 10)

- Popliteus (chapter 14)

- Soleus/Plantaris: see plantaris (chapter 16)

- Gastrocnemius (chapter 15)

- Adductor Muscles of the Hip (chapter 11)

Conclusion

You may also need to search the piriformis, gluteus medius, posterior portion of the gluteus minimus, vastus lateralis (quadriceps femoris), popliteus, gastrocnemius, and plantaris muscles since trigger points in those muscles can cause similar pain referral patterns. Since trigger points in the piriformis and gluteus medius muscles don't directly cause lower leg, knee, ankle, or foot pain, they are not addressed in this book. If you can't relieve your pain with the self-help techniques in this book within six to eight weeks, you may wish to consider whether you need to treat trigger points in these other muscles. See the Resources section for books and other resources that can provide guidance on self-treatment of muscles not covered in this book.

Tight hamstrings will tend to cause a flattened lumbar spine and a head-forward posture, resulting in problems in a number of muscles not covered in this book: the quadratus lumborum (lumbar area), paraspinals, iliopsoas, rectus abdominis (abdominal), posterior neck, pectoralis minor (upper chest), infraspinatus (back of shoulder blade), subscapularis (front of shoulder blade), teres minor (between shoulder blade and upper humerus bone), and supraspinatus (above the shoulder blade) muscles. You should search these muscles for trigger points, particularly if you have upper-body symptoms that are only temporarily relieved. (See chapter 4, Body Mechanics, for more information on head-forward posture and also see the Resources section.)

You may get misdiagnosed with sciatica, since the pain from sciatica is similar to that of hamstrings trigger points. You may need to see a health care provider to rule out osteoarthritis of the knee. Misalignment of the sacroiliac joint and L4-5 and L5-S1 vertebrae can cause spasm and restriction of the hamstrings muscles. See a chiropractor or osteopathic physician for evaluation and treatment.

Chapter 14

Popliteus

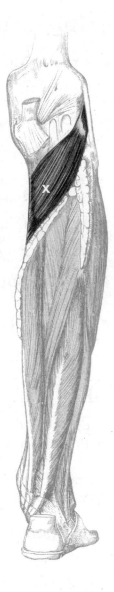

Common Symptoms

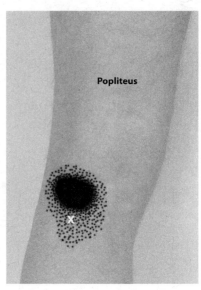

Popliteus

- Trigger points refer pain to the back of the knee when you are crouching, running, or walking, and pain is worse when you walk down stairs or downhill.

- You may have knee pain when straightening your leg.

- Trigger points are usually found after trigger points in the gastrocnemius or biceps femoris have been inactivated.

- You may have a slight decrease in range of motion, which may be unnoticeable.

Possible Causes and Perpetuators

Injuries or Muscle Abuse

- Playing sports that require you to twist, slide, and change direction suddenly, such as soccer, football, and baseball

- Running or skiing downhill

- Receiving a trauma or strain that tears the posterior cruciate ligament (a ligament in the knee joint that connects the tibia to the femur)

- Tearing the plantaris muscle in the calf

Medical or Structural

- Foot pronation, especially combined with activities listed in previous section

Helpful Hints

If you do any of the sports activities listed above, you may need to condition this muscle gradually with the help of a physical therapist. Gradually add distance to your runs or hikes rather than suddenly increasing the mileage. Avoid running or walking on side-slanted surfaces, or at least change directions periodically so you are running on the opposite slant.

Prior to doing an aggravating activity, take extra vitamin C, and be sure to keep your legs warm.

Do not wear high heels. Get corrective orthotics to correct foot pronation problems.

Self-Help Techniques

Caution: Do not apply pressure to your legs if you have varicose veins in the area to be treated—it could release a clot that could go to your heart or brain! *An acupuncturist or massage therapist should treat your legs, because they can avoid the veins.*

Applying Pressure

Do the gastrocnemius self-work first (chapter 15), being careful to work close to but not into the back crease of the knee.

Popliteus Pressure

Sit in a chair and bend forward slightly, supporting yourself with one hand on a thigh. *Don't press into the crease behind the knee—there are veins and nerves that are close to the surface.* But do get close to it, because the bulk of the muscle is on the inside of the knee. To work on this part of the muscle, use your thumb of the opposite hand. To work on the part of the muscle closer to the outside of your knee, use the hand on the same side. If you keep your thumb straight, it is easier to press through the overlying muscles into the trigger points in the popliteus. You may need the help of a massage therapist if you have a hard time reaching this area.

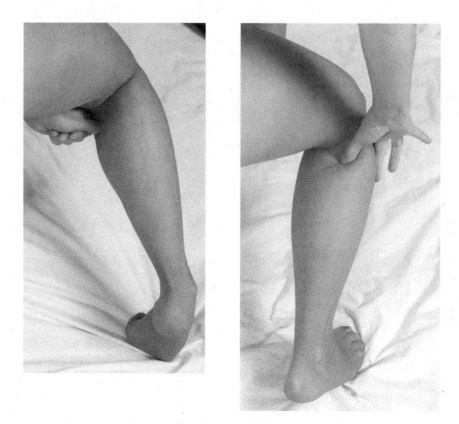

Also See

- Quadriceps Femoris: see biceps femoris (chapter 10)

- Gastrocnemius (chapter 15)

Conclusion

Remember that trigger points in the popliteus muscle are usually found after trigger points in the gastrocnemius or biceps femoris have been inactivated, so you will want to be sure to work on those muscles.

Chapter 15

Gastrocnemius

The Achilles tendon attaches the gastrocnemius and soleus muscles to the heel bone. If the tendon feels tight, work on the muscle bellies to relax the tendon.

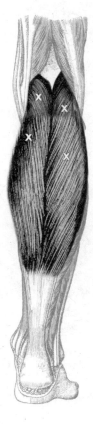

Common Symptoms

- Trigger points refer pain into the arch of your foot, over the back of your leg, to the back of your knee, and possibly to the back of your lower thigh.

- You may have pain with climbing steep slopes, climbing over rocks, or walking on slanted surfaces. You probably have difficulty walking fast, and a tendency to walk with a flat-footed, stiff-legged gait. You may have difficulty straightening your leg completely when standing.

- You may have calf cramps when sleeping.

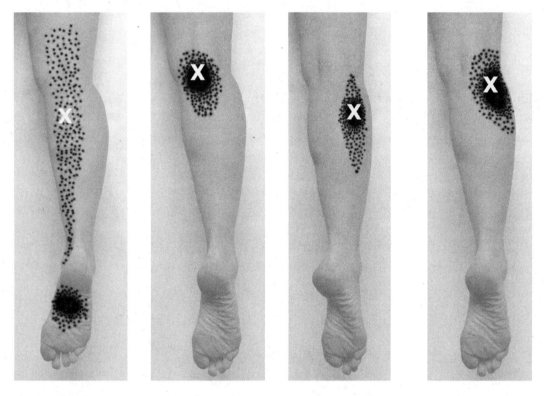

Gastrocnemius

Possible Causes and Perpetuators

Postural

- Prolonged immobility with your toes pointed, such as when sleeping

- Riding a bicycle with the seat too low

- Standing while leaning forward for a prolonged time

- Hooking your heel on a rung of a stool for a prolonged time

- Driving a car with an accelerator pedal that is too horizontal

- Sitting in a chair with a high front edge that impairs circulation or otherwise compresses the backs of your thighs

- Sitting in a reclining chair that places a lot of your leg weight on your calves

- Squatting for long periods

Injuries or Muscle Abuse

- Walking, climbing, or running up steep slopes, over rocks, or on slanted surfaces

- Wearing socks, garters, or knee-high hose with an elastic band that is too tight

- Wearing high heels

Medical or Structural

- Impaired circulation

- Wearing a cast

- Viral infections

Other

- Muscle chilling

Helpful Hints

Calf cramps are one of the most common symptoms of gastrocnemius trigger points, and often occur when sleeping or sitting for too long with your toes pointed. If this happens, rather than standing and walking immediately, instead gently flex your foot so that your toes are moving toward your knees, and then release. Keep your calves and body warm. Use a space heater near your legs if necessary. To reduce the tendency for your calves to cramp when sleeping, keep them warm at night by using a heating pad at bedtime, or use an electric blanket. Sleep with a warm covering on your legs, such as knee-high pile socks or long johns. Please see "Calf Cramping" in chapter 3 for additional self-help techniques.

At night, place a pillow against the bottom of your feet to maintain a 90-degree angle between your feet and lower leg. Avoid hooking your heels on the rung of a stool. Sit in a chair at the proper height for you so it doesn't restrict circulation in the back of your thighs, and use a slanted footstool to elevate the lower legs if necessary. Using a rocking chair prevents prolonged immobility and increases circulation. If you swim, avoid the crawl stroke, since the kick causes you to point your toes.

Don't wear high heels, and avoid wearing smooth-leather–soled shoes, particularly on a slippery floor. If your socks or hose leave a mark or indentation on your skin at the elastic band, the elastic is too tight and is cutting off needed circulation. Buy socks and hose with a wider, looser band.

Until the trigger points are inactivated, avoid walking up hills or on slanted surfaces. Stretch before and after athletic activities.

See "Compartment Syndromes" in chapter 3. If you have a compartment syndrome, *it is important to see a doctor immediately for treatment.*

Self-Help Techniques

Caution: Do not apply pressure to your legs if you have varicose veins in the area to be treated—it could release a clot that could go to your heart or brain! *An acupuncturist or massage therapist should treat your legs, because they can avoid the veins.* You may still do the stretches below.

Applying Pressure

Gastrocnemius/Soleus Pressure

Lie face up with your butt scooted up close to a chair, coffee table, or other hard surface that is about the height you need to get a 90-degree-angle bend at your knee. Place a therapy ball on the hard surface and rest your calf on it, with gravity giving you the needed pressure. Be sure to work as much as you can top to bottom, and rotate your leg side to side to get as much of the edges of the muscles as you can. You can move your leg over the ball (following the guidelines in chapter 7), and you will also need to move the ball with your hand at least once to get to the entire muscle.

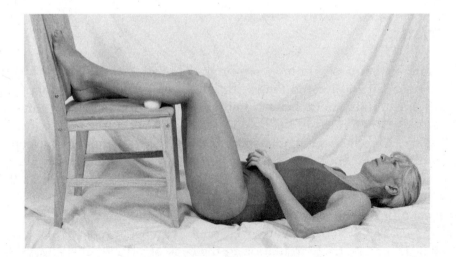

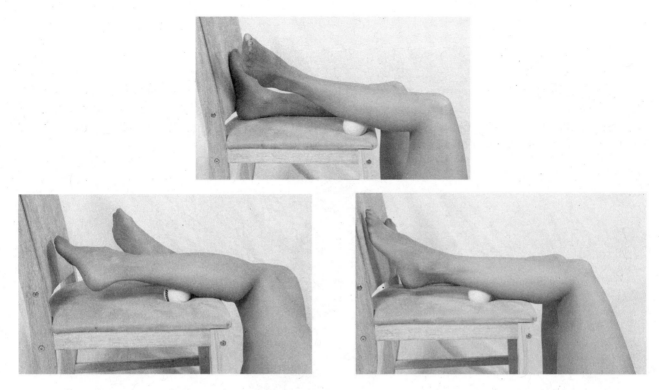

Then sit up with your legs bent to one side. Using a golf ball, tennis ball, or other pressure device in the center of your palm, press into tender points on your inner and outer lower legs to work the edges of the muscles.

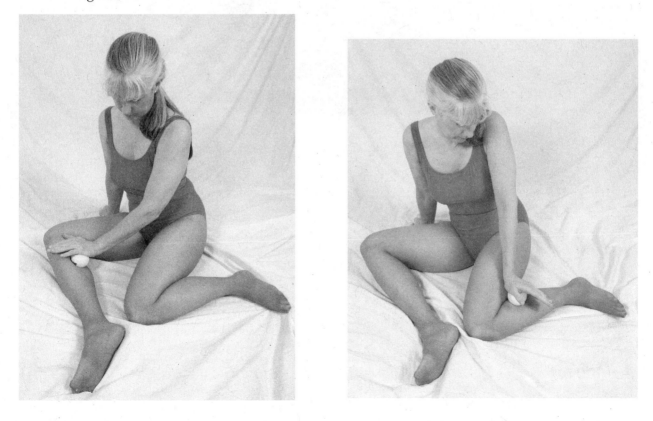

Stretches

Gastrocnemius Stretch

Stand a short distance from a wall, and place your hands on the wall at about head height. Stretch one leg out behind you, with the knee straight, the heel on the floor, and the toes pointing straight forward. Let your hips move forward until you are getting a gentle stretch on the back of the lower leg. Look straight ahead so your neck is not bent down.

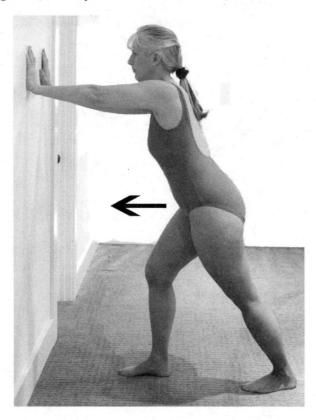

Exercises

Seated Gastrocnemius Stretch/Conditioning

Sit with your back against a wall with your legs out straight, and put a thin, long towel around one foot and hold both ends with your hands. Gently press the ball of your foot against the towel for five seconds, while you slowly inhale. As you exhale, release the pressure on your foot and use the towel to pull the ball of the foot toward you, giving you a gentle stretch on the back of the calf. Repeat three or four times with each foot.

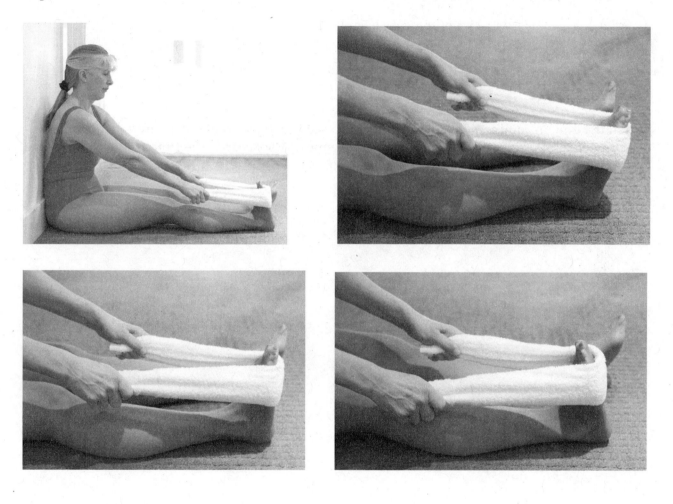

Also See

- Soleus/Plantaris: see soleus (chapter 16)

- Hamstrings (chapter 13)

- Gluteus Minimus: see posterior portion (chapter 9)

- Tibialis Anterior (chapter 19)

- Long Extensor Muscles of the Toes (chapter 21)

Conclusion

Search the gluteus minimus (posterior portion) to see if trigger points there are causing and perpetuating satellite trigger points in the gastrocnemius. Also, search the tibialis anterior and the long extensors of the toes for associated trigger points.

Chapter 16

Soleus/Plantaris

The soleus muscle is known as the body's "second heart," due to its pumping action that returns blood from the lower leg to the heart. Flexing and extending your foot can greatly improve circulation in your legs.

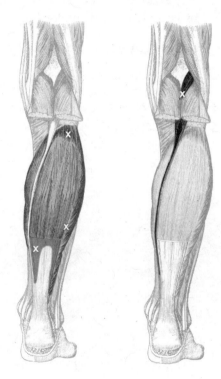

Common Symptoms

- Trigger points in both muscles cause you to be unable to flex your foot toward your knee, making it difficult to squat or kneel down to pick items up off the floor, which can subsequently lead to back pain due to improper lifting.

- You may have difficulty walking due to pain, especially uphill and up or down stairs.

Soleus Trigger Points

- The most common trigger point in the soleus muscle refers pain to the back and bottom of your heel, and the Achilles tendon.

- The second most common trigger point in the soleus muscle is located close to the back of your knee and refers pain to the upper half of the back of your calf.

- An uncommon trigger point refers pain over your sacroiliac joint on the same side.

- Trigger points in the soleus muscle may be the cause of "growing pains" in children.

- Trigger points and subsequent tightness of the soleus muscle can entrap the posterior tibial veins, posterior tibial artery, and tibial nerve, causing swelling of your foot and ankle and severe heel pain and tingling.

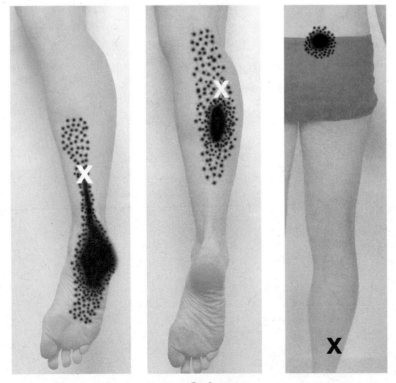

Soleus

Plantaris Trigger Points

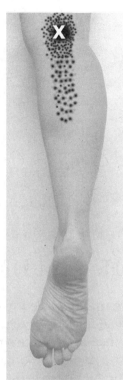

- Trigger points in the plantaris muscle refer pain behind your knee and to the upper half of your calf.

- A tight plantaris muscle can entrap the popliteal artery, which can cause calf pain.

Plantaris

Possible Causes and Perpetuators

Postural

- Sitting in a chair that is too high, so that you are not able to keep your feet flat on the ground; sitting in a chair with a high front edge that impairs circulation or otherwise compresses the back of your thighs; or sitting in a reclining chair that puts a lot of the leg weight on your calves

- Prolonged immobility with your toes pointed, such as when sleeping

- Prolonged squatting

Injuries or Muscle Abuse

- Running/jogging

- A direct blow to the muscle

- A fall or near-fall

- Wearing high heels, smooth-soled shoes on slippery surfaces, or shoes that are too stiff

- Wearing socks or knee-high hose with an elastic band that is too tight

- Skiing or ice skating without stiff boots

- Walking, climbing, or running up steep slopes, over rocks, or on slanted surfaces, especially when you are not used to it

- Sustained pressure against the calf

Medical or Structural

- Having one leg anatomically shorter than the other, since the short side bears more of the body weight

Other

- Referral from trigger points in the gluteus minimus muscle (posterior portion)

- Chilling of your calf, especially combined with immobility

Helpful Hints

At night, place a pillow against the bottom of your feet to maintain a 90-degree angle between your feet and lower leg. If you sleep on your back, try putting a small pillow under your knees. Wear knee-high fleece socks at night to prevent muscle chilling.

Avoid hooking your heels on the rung of a stool. Sit in a chair at the proper height for you so that it doesn't restrict circulation in the back of your thighs, and use a slanted footstool to elevate your lower legs, if necessary. Using a rocking chair prevents prolonged immobility and increases circulation. Most recliner chairs or footrests place too much pressure on the calf; if you choose to use some kind of lower leg support, make sure you get something that supports the whole back of the lower leg and heels so that no one area takes all the weight of the leg. When driving for long periods, take frequent breaks and use cruise control.

Don't wear high heels, and avoid wearing smooth-leather–soled shoes, particularly on slippery floors. If your shoes are so stiff that they don't bend at the toes very well, you will need to find more pliable shoes. Proper shoes are so important to lasting relief of soleus trigger points that if you are unwilling to change your shoes, you can expect to need frequent treatment. If your socks or hose leave a mark or indentation on your skin at the elastic band, the elastic is too tight and is cutting off needed circulation. Buy socks and hose with a wider, looser band. If you have one leg shorter than the other, you will need to see a specialist for compensating lifts.

Until your trigger points are inactivated, avoid walking up hills or on slanted surfaces. If you have pain with walking up stairs, try rotating your body to 45 degrees (instead of facing forward), keep your body erect, and put your entire foot on the next step, rather than letting your heel hang off of the edge. Stretch before and after athletic activities. If you swim, avoid the crawl stroke, since the kick causes you to point your toes.

If you have heel pain and a bone spur is found on the bottom of the big bone of the heel, don't assume the spur is the source of the pain. The other heel may have a spur that causes no pain, so trigger points, rather than the spur, may be the source of the pain. An elevated serum uric acid level will cause a heel spur to become painful and is likely to aggravate trigger points in the soleus and other muscles. (See "Heel Spurs" in chapter 3 for more information.)

An Achilles tendinopathy (formerly called tendinitis) may be due to trigger points causing shortening of the soleus and gastrocnemius muscles. Pain will be diffuse and possibly burning in or around the Achilles tendon, and aggravated by activity. If the condition is severe, there also may be swelling, crackling sounds, or a tender nodule in the tendon. The cause is usually improper training or too much training. Corrective orthotics and shoes with a more flexible sole may help considerably. (See "Achilles Tendinopathy and Ruptures" in chapter 3 for more information.)

Also see "Compartment Syndromes" in chapter 3. In the case of the soleus muscle, a compartment syndrome is called *soleus periostalgia syndrome*. This is caused by repetitive exercise, such as running or aerobic dancing. The membrane over the surface of the bone (*periosteum*) where the soleus attaches on the inside of the lower leg can be loosened and sometimes separated from the deeper part of the bone. A stress fracture can cause similar symptoms. If you have a compartment syndrome, *it is important to see a doctor immediately for treatment.*

Self-Help Techniques

Caution: Do not apply pressure to your legs if you have varicose veins in the area to be treated—it could release a clot that could go to your heart or brain! *An acupuncturist or massage therapist should treat your legs, because they can avoid the veins.* You may still do the stretch below.

Applying Pressure

Soleus/Gastrocnemius Pressure

The self-help pressure is the same for both muscles (see chapter 15).

Stretches

Soleus Stretch

Hold onto something for support. Place one foot out in front of you and one foot slightly behind you, with the toes of both feet pointing straight forward. Keeping your heel on the floor, bend the knee of the forward leg until you are getting a gentle stretch in the soleus muscle. Look straight ahead so that your neck is not bent down.

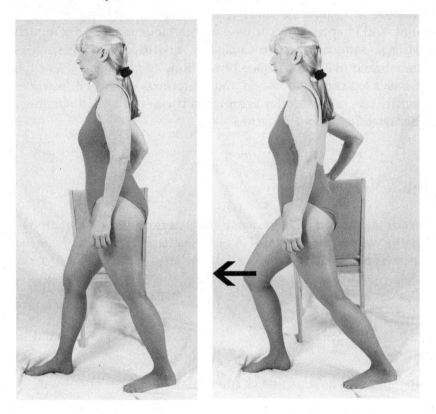

Also See

- Deep Intrinsic Foot Muscles: see quadratus plantae (chapter 23)

- Superficial Intrinsic Foot Muscles: see abductor hallucis (chapter 22)

- Gastrocnemius (chapter 15)

- Tibialis Posterior (chapter 17)

- Long Flexor Muscles of the Toes (chapter 20)

- Tibialis Anterior (chapter 19)

- Long Extensor Muscles of the Toes (chapter 21)

- Peroneal Muscles: peroneus tertius (chapter 18)

Conclusion

Search for trigger points in the quadratus plantae, since it can also cause pain on the bottom of your heel. If you have trigger points in the soleus and also have knee pain, search for trigger points in the quadriceps femoris, since loss of function in the calf puts additional stress on the front-of-the-thigh muscles.

Chapter 17

Tibialis Posterior

The tibialis posterior muscle is located in between the bones of the lower leg. It attaches to both the tibia and fibula on the sides, and its tendon attaches to several bones in the bottom of the foot, functioning to help distribute body weight evenly on the sole of the foot. Weakness or absence of this muscle causes severe pronation, leading to breakdown of one of the arches of the foot and subsequent severe deformity. Any problems must be corrected within a few months to prevent permanent damage. You will need the help of a professional to treat this muscle, but because tibialis posterior trigger points rarely occur alone, by treating the trigger points in other associated muscles, you can greatly speed your treatment and healing and help prevent permanent damage.

Doctors Travell and Simons nicknamed trigger points in the tibialis posterior muscle "Runner's Nemesis," since running on uneven surfaces is the most common contributor to activation and perpetuation. Obesity, hypertension, lupus, diabetes, peripheral neuropathy, smoking, gout, and rheumatoid arthritis are also predisposing factors to problems in the tibialis posterior muscle and tendon.

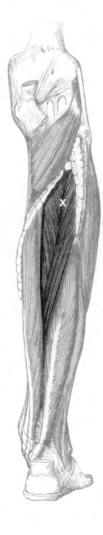

Common Symptoms

- Trigger points refer pain primarily over your Achilles' tendon, with spillover pain through your heel, to the bottom of your foot and toes, and over the back of your calf.

- You probably have pain in the foot when running or walking, especially on uneven surfaces.

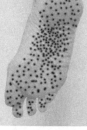

Tibialis posterior

Possible Causes and Perpetuators

Injuries or Muscle Abuse

- Running or jogging, especially on uneven ground or side-slanted surfaces

- Shoes that are worn down on the inside or outside edges

Medical or Structural

- Foot pronation

- Having a longer second toe (causing an unstable ankle and foot rocking)

- Hyperuricemia with or without symptoms of gout in the big toe (diagnosed with a blood test)

- Polymyalgia rheumatica (diagnosed with a blood test)

Helpful Hints

Get good orthotics with arch support and a deep heel cup to prevent pronation. Avoid high heels and shoes that don't fit properly.

Walk or run only on smooth, level surfaces until trigger points are inactivated. If you are unable to walk or run, try swimming and bicycling.

See "Shin Splints and Tibial Periosteal Stress Syndromes" in chapter 3. In the case of the tibialis posterior muscle, shin splints usually develop in runners who are novices and athletes who are poorly conditioned. The surface of the bone (periosteum) where the tibialis posterior attaches on the tibia can be loosened and sometimes separated from the deeper part of the bone.

See "Compartment Syndromes" in chapter 3. If you have a compartment syndrome, *it is important to see a doctor immediately for treatment.*

Self-Help Techniques

Caution: Do not apply pressure to your legs if you have varicose veins in the area to be treated—it could release a clot that could go to your heart or brain! *An acupuncturist or massage therapist should treat your legs, because they can avoid the veins.*

Applying Pressure

The tibialis posterior is deep and next to the bone, so you may not be able to get to the whole muscle with self-help techniques. Try using the gastrocnemius pressure self-help technique in chapter 15. Ultrasound and stretching, with the help of a physical therapist or other qualified professional, are effective.

Also See

- Long Flexor Muscles of the Toes (chapter 20)

- Peroneal Muscles: see peroneus longus, peroneus brevis (chapter 18)

Conclusion

If a tight tibialis posterior is not treated, the tendon can become elongated, accompanied by severe pain with walking and displacement of the bones of the foot. The tendon can also rupture. This requires diagnosis by an MRI.

Chapter 18

Peroneal Muscle Group

The upper portions of the peroneus longus, brevis, and tertius attach to the fibula, with their tendons attaching on bones in the foot. Weakness of any of the three peroneal muscles can contribute to "weak ankles," causing frequent ankle sprains and making you prone to ankle fractures, which then further perpetuates trigger points. Treatment of peroneal muscle trigger points is critical to breaking this self-perpetuating cycle.

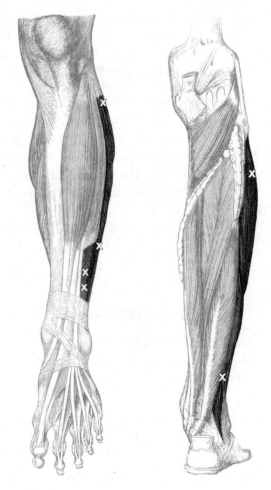

Common Symptoms

- Trigger points in the peroneus longus and brevis muscles refer pain and tenderness over and around your outside ankle bone, over a small area on the outside of your foot, and possibly over a small area over the outside of your lower leg.

- Trigger points in the peroneus tertius muscle refer pain and tenderness more toward the front of your ankle and possibly behind your outside ankle bone and down over your heel.

- You may have weak ankles, which are easily broken or sprained over the outside of the ankle.

- You may have difficulty with in-line or ice skating, unless the boots are very stiff.

- If the deep peroneal nerve is entrapped, you may trip frequently due to an inability to lift your foot.

- Because of the tenderness and pain in and around your ankle joint, trigger point referral can be misdiagnosed by a health care provider as arthritis.

- Entrapment of the common peroneal nerve, superficial peroneal nerve, or deep peroneal nerve can cause pain and odd sensations (such as numbness) of the front of the ankle and foot, accompanied by weakness of your ankle.

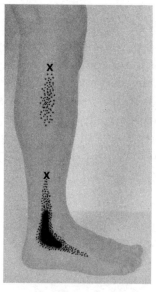 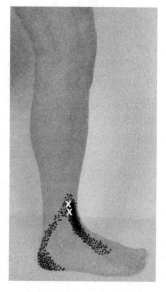

**Peroneus longus
(upper)
Peroneus brevis
(lower)**

Peroneus tertius

Possible Causes and Perpetuators

Postural

- Crossing one leg over the other, which can compress the common peroneal nerve

- Sleeping with your toes pointed

- Wearing high heels or shoes with a spike heel of any height

Injuries or Muscle Abuse

- Wearing socks or knee-high hose with an elastic band that is too tight

- Referred pain from trigger points in the gluteus minimus muscle (anterior portion)

- Associated trigger points in the tibialis anterior and tibialis posterior muscles

Medical or Structural

- Sprains or fractures in the lower leg, ankle, or foot

- Immobilization with a cast

- Having a longer second toe

- Having one leg anatomically shorter than the other

Helpful Hints

If your socks or hose leave a mark or indentation on your skin from the elastic band, the elastic is too tight and is cutting off needed circulation. Buy socks and hose with a wider, looser band.

Don't wear spiked or high heels. Avoid shoes with pointed toes and inadequate room across the top of the toes. Your feet get wider as you get older, and shoes that may once have fit properly may now be too narrow. Any shoes that don't fit or are worn unevenly on the bottoms should be discarded. Buy shoes that have wide soles, such as athletic shoes, and get orthotic inserts with a deep heel cup and good arch support (most shoes made these days have minimal or no arch support). If your foot supinates due to a longer second toe (you will see excessive wear on the outside edge of the heel of your shoe), you will need to get corrective orthotics.

Walk or run on smooth, level surfaces until trigger points are relieved. Avoid slanted sidewalks, roads, or tracks.

Crossing one leg over the other to compensate for a small hemipelvis (see page 40) can compress the common peroneal nerve. If one leg is shorter than the other, you may have pain on only one side, even if you have a longer second toe on both sides. This is because your weight is shifted to the shorter side, causing a chronic overload of the muscles on that side. The leg may be "shorter" due to foot pronation and a low arch on the affected side rather than an anatomically unequal leg bone length. You will need to see a specialist for corrective orthotics or compensating lifts and pads for any of these conditions.

If you have pain remaining after a broken leg, ankle, or foot, try searching for trigger points in these muscles, since immobilization with a cast will cause trigger points.

Read "Compartment Syndromes" in chapter 3. If you have this condition, *it is important to see a doctor for treatment immediately.*

Self-Help Techniques

Caution: Do not apply pressure to your legs if you have varicose veins in the area to be treated—it could release a clot that could go to your heart or brain! *An acupuncturist or massage therapist should treat your legs, because they can avoid the veins.* You may still do the stretch below.

Search the gluteus minimus (chapter 9) for trigger points first (anterior portion, on the side under your pants seam), since trigger points in that muscle can activate and perpetuate trigger points in the peroneal muscles.

Applying Pressure

Peroneal Muscle Pressure

Lie on your side on your bed, with a tennis ball between the bed and the side of your lower leg, using gravity for pressure. You can move your leg over the ball to reposition it. If you want more pressure, you can rest the top leg on the lower leg.

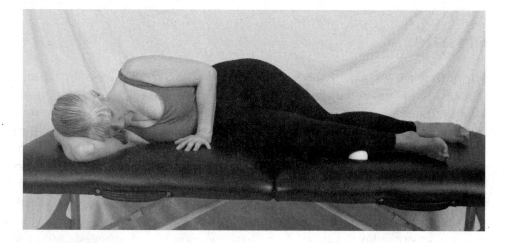

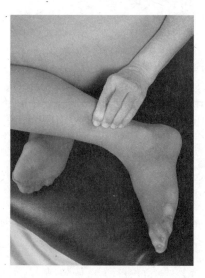

Then sit up with your leg out to the side on the bed, and use your fingers to check for trigger points in the peroneus tertius, one to two inches above the outside ankle bone and closer toward the front of the leg.

Stretches

Peroneal Stretch

To stretch the right peroneal muscles, bring your right foot close to your left thigh or on top of it, depending on how flexible you are. Use your hands to rotate your foot so the bottom is toward the ceiling. Now flex that foot so you are bringing the toes toward your right knee. You should feel the stretch on the outside of your lower leg. Repeat with the other leg. You may also do this stretch in a hot bath.

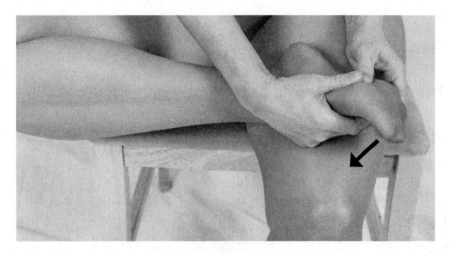

Also See

- Gluteus Minimus: see anterior portion (chapter 9)

- Tibialis Anterior (chapter 19)

- Tibialis Posterior (chapter 17)

- Long Extensor Muscles of the Toes: see extensor digitorum longus (chapter 21)

Conclusion

Be sure to also search for trigger points in the gluteus minimus, tibialis anterior, and tibialis posterior muscles, since they often cause secondary trigger points to form in the peroneal muscles.

Chapter 19

Tibialis Anterior

The tibialis anterior attaches to the tibia on the front of the lower leg, and runs from the knee area down to its tendon attachments on some of the bones in the foot. Proper function of this muscle is essential for walking and sports activities, because it moves your toes up out of the way as you take each step. If you are elderly, trigger points in this muscle can be of particular concern because of the associated risks of falling due to balance problems and tripping.

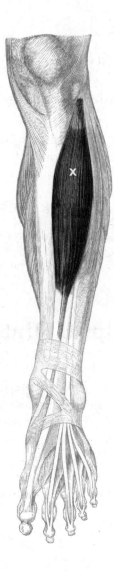

Common Symptoms

- Trigger points refer pain over the front of your ankle and the top and side of your big toe, and possibly over the front of your lower leg and top of your foot.

- Trigger points usually occur in combination with trigger points in other leg muscles.

- You may have ankle weakness or pain with motion.

- You are probably unable to lift your toes up out of the way when walking, causing you to trip or fall.

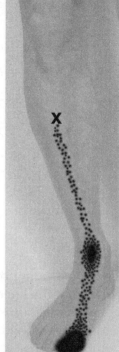

Possible Causes and Perpetuators

Injuries or Muscle Abuse

- Experiencing a direct trauma to the muscle, as in a direct blow or some other force severe enough to cause a sprained ankle or broken bone

- Walking on rough ground or a slanted surface

- Catching a toe on an object while walking

- Hiking in the spring after walking on level surfaces all winter

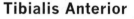

Tibialis Anterior

Helpful Hints

If your foot pronates (you will see excessive wear on the inside edge of the sole of your shoe), you will need to get corrective orthotics.

If the accelerator pedal in your car is at a steep vertical angle, try putting a wedge on the pedal with the big end at the bottom to reduce the angle of your foot. If it is nearly horizontal, try putting the big end of the wedge at the top. Using cruise control will help. Take breaks every thirty to sixty minutes.

At night, place a pillow against the bottom of your feet to maintain a 90-degree angle between your feet and lower leg.

Walk on smooth, level surfaces until trigger points are relieved. Then start adding short hills to strengthen the muscle. You can start adding distance slowly, trying to stay within a range where the muscle does not get sore afterward.

Read "Shin Splints and Tibial Periosteal Stress Syndromes" in chapter 3. Trigger points in the tibialis anterior can cause tibial periosteal stress, which is sometimes called "anterior shin splints."

Read "Compartment Syndromes" in chapter 3. If you have a compartment syndrome, *it is important to see a doctor for treatment immediately.*

Self-Help Techniques

Caution: Do not apply pressure to your legs if you have varicose veins in the area to be treated— it could release a clot that could go to your heart or brain! *An acupuncturist or massage therapist should treat your legs, because they can avoid the veins.* You may still do the stretches below.

It is essential to do self-help techniques on the calves first, since tightness in those muscles is likely the cause of trigger points in the tibialis anterior. If you release the tibialis anterior first, it could make the pain in the front of the leg much worse. See the soleus/gastrocnemius pressure technique and stretches in chapters 15 and 16.

Applying Pressure

Tibialis Anterior Pressure

Even though most trigger points will be found in the upper third of the tibialis anterior, I like to work the entire length of the muscle. Get down on the floor on all fours, and place the tennis ball under the front of your lower leg. The weight of your leg should give you enough pressure. If you need more or less pressure, shift your weight toward or away from the side you are working on. Be sure to keep your head relaxed and let it hang down.

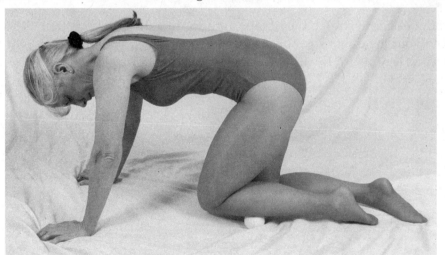

Stretches

Tibialis Anterior Stretch

Cross your leg over the opposite thigh, and pull your foot and toes back toward you with your hand so you feel a stretch on the front of your leg. Moving your toes toward the ceiling or the floor will give you a slightly different stretch, so explore which angle is best for you.

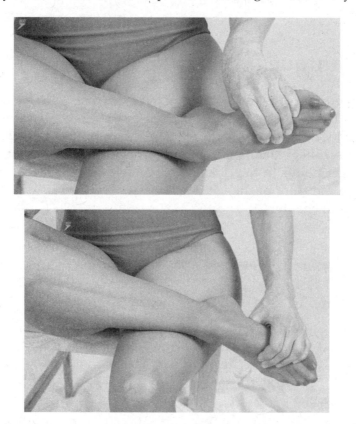

You may find it easier to stretch the tibialis anterior in a different position: Scoot to the edge of a chair, and drop your leg down so your toe is pointing behind you and the top of your foot is on the floor. Press your leg toward the floor until you get a gentle stretch.

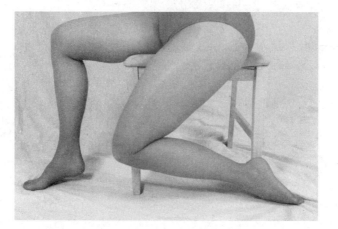

Also See

- Long Extensor Muscles of the Toes (chapter 21)

- Superficial Intrinsic Foot Muscles: see extensor digitorum brevis, extensor hallucis brevis (chapter 22)

- Peroneal Muscles: see peroneus tertius, peroneus longus (chapter 18)

- Long Flexor Muscles of the Toes: see flexor hallucis longus (chapter 20)

- Deep Intrinsic Foot Muscles: see first interosseous (chapter 23)

Conclusion

Since trigger points in many other leg muscles can have similar referral patterns, be sure to also search for trigger points in the long extensors of toes (extensor hallucis longus, extensor digitorum longus), superficial intrinsic foot muscles (extensor digitorum brevis, extensor hallucis brevis), peroneal muscles (peroneus tertius and longus), long flexor muscles of toes (flexor hallucis longus), and deep intrinsic foot muscles (first interosseous).

If you find trigger points in the tibialis anterior, there will also likely be trigger points in the peroneus longus (peroneal), and possibly the extensor digitorum longus and extensor hallucis longus (long extensors of toes).

Chapter 20

Long Flexor Muscles of the Toes

Hammer toes and claw toes can form when the long flexor muscles of the toes attempt to compensate for a flat foot (pronation). They can also form when the gastrocnemius and soleus muscles are weak (causing the outside and deeper rear calf muscles to try to compensate) combined with a high arch and foot supination, but this is less common.

Tightness and trigger points in the flexor hallucis longus can cause hallux valgus, which was discussed in chapter 3 under "Bunions and Hallux Valgus."

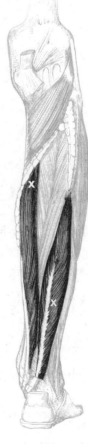

Common Symptoms

- Trigger points in the flexor digitorum longus muscle refer pain primarily to the front half of the arch of your foot and into the ball of your foot, and sometimes also into the second through fifth toes, and very occasionally over the inside of your calf and ankle area.

- Trigger points in the flexor hallucis longus refer pain to the bottom of your big toe and the ball of your foot adjacent to your big toe.

- You probably have pain when walking.

- Trigger points may occasionally cause painful cramping similar to gastrocnemius cramps.

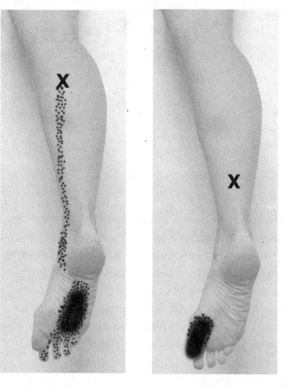

Flexor digitorum longus   **Flexor hallucis longus**

Possible Causes and Perpetuators

Injuries or Muscle Abuse

- Walking, running, or jogging on uneven ground, sand, or side-slanted surfaces

- Wearing shoes with worn soles and reduced cushioning, or wearing shoes that aren't very flexible

Medical or Structural

- Foot pronation

- Having a longer second toe (causing an unstable ankle and foot rocking)

- Having weak gastrocnemius and soleus muscles combined with a high arch and foot supination

Helpful Hints

Wear comfortable shoes with flexible soles and good shock absorption, and make sure they don't cramp the toes, and that the heels aren't too loose. Replace worn shoes, and don't wear high heels. If your ankle is *hypomobile* (doesn't have much movement), see a chiropractor or osteopathic physician to increase mobility. If it is *hypermobile* (moves too much), orthotics with good arch support and a deep heel cup, along with ankle-high shoes for support, will help stabilize your foot.

Until trigger points are inactivated, walk or run only on smooth surfaces, start with short distances, and increase mileage gradually. Try rowing, swimming, or bicycling instead.

Read "Shin Splints and Tibial Periosteal Stress Syndromes" in chapter 3. Trigger points in the long toe flexor muscles can cause medial tibial stress syndrome. The flexor digitorum longus attachment on the inside of the lower leg can be loosened and sometimes separated from the deeper part of the bone. A stress fracture can cause similar symptoms.

Read "Compartment Syndromes" in chapter 3. If you have a compartment syndrome, *it is important to see a doctor for treatment immediately.*

Self-Help Techniques

Caution: Do not apply pressure to your legs if you have varicose veins in the area to be treated—it could release a clot that could go to your heart or brain! *An acupuncturist or massage therapist should treat your legs, because they can avoid the veins.* You may still do the stretch and exercises below.

Applying Pressure

The gastrocnemius self-work (chapter 15) will also benefit the long flexor muscles of the toes.

Stretches

Long Toe Flexors Stretch

In a seated position, rest your heel on a stool or the floor with your ankle flexed back toward your body. With the fingers of one hand, pull the toes of one foot toward you. Then slowly press those toes away from you, against the fingers of the hand you are using to pull the toes toward you. Relax, and repeat.

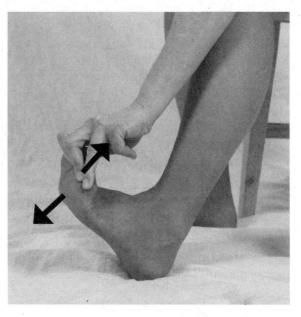

Exercises

Walk in a swimming pool in waist-deep water, taking long strides.

Also See

- Tibialis posterior (chapter 17)

- Superficial Intrinsic Foot Muscles (chapter 22)

- Deep Intrinsic Foot Muscles: see adductor hallucis, interossei, flexor hallucis brevis (chapter 23)

- Long Extensor Muscles of the Toes (chapter 21)

Conclusion

Also search for trigger points in the tibialis posterior, superficial intrinsic foot muscles (abductor digiti minimi, flexor digitorum brevis), and deep intrinsic foot muscles (adductor hallucis, interossei, flexor hallucis brevis), since they have similar referral patterns.

The tendon of the flexor hallucis longus can rupture spontaneously with overload, without previous injury or disease, and must be repaired surgically.

Chapter 21

Long Extensor Muscles of the Toes

Chronic tension of the long extensors of the toes can lead to hammer toe, claw toe, or mallet toe. Chronic tension in the flexor digitorum longus and/or weakness in the *lumbricals* (deep muscles on the bottom of the foot) can cause pain in the foot, leading you to lift your foot in a flat manner to avoid forefoot pressure, which overloads the extensor digitorum longus muscle. Wearing tight shoes can cause the lumbricals to atrophy or to fail to develop normally during childhood.

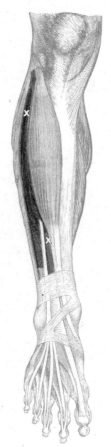

Common Symptoms

- Trigger points in the extensor digitorum longus refer pain mainly to the top of your foot and over the tops of the three middle toes, and sometimes over the front of your ankle and lower half of the front of the lower leg.

- Trigger points in the extensor hallucis longus refer pain over the top of the foot close to your big toe, over the top of your big toe, and sometimes over your ankle and a little onto the front of your lower leg.

- When you are walking, the ball of the foot slaps down after heel strike, or your foot will feel "weak."

- Trigger points can cause cramps at night in the front of your lower leg when it is fatigued or when your toes are flexed toward the kneecaps for a prolonged period.

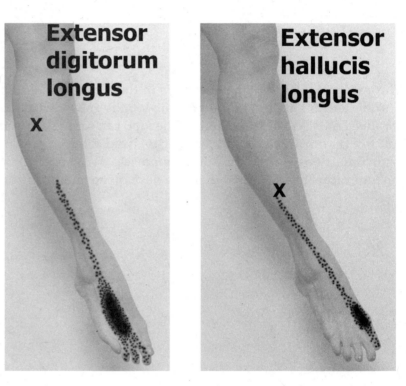

Extensor digitorum longus

Extensor hallucis longus

- Trigger points can cause "growing pains" in children and adolescents.

- A tight extensor digitorum longus muscle can entrap the deep peroneal nerve and cause weakness in the muscles on the front of your lower leg and an inability to control the upward movement of your forefoot.

Possible Causes and Perpetuators

Injuries or Muscle Abuse

- Tripping or falling

- A direct trauma to the muscle

- Catching a toe on the ground when kicking a ball

- Driving a car with an accelerator pedal that is too vertical or too horizontal

- Sitting in a chair with your feet tucked back a bit

- Wearing high heels

- Tight gastrocnemius and/or soleus muscles which lead to a tight Achilles' tendon, restricting foot movement

- Unaccustomed excessive walking, jogging, or running, especially on uneven ground

- Sleeping with your toes pointed

Medical or Structural

- A nerve root irritation at the L-4 or L-5 vertebra

- A stress fracture in one of the bones of the lower leg

- Wearing a cast after a fracture, or immobilization after a sprain

- Anterior compartment syndrome (see chapter 19, Tibialis Anterior)

- Nutritional problems (see chapter 5)

Helpful Hints

Wear low heels or flat shoes with a wide base, and get some good orthotics. If your ankle is *hypomobile* (doesn't have much movement), see a chiropractor or osteopathic physician to increase mobility. If it is *hypermobile* (moves too much), orthotics with good arch support and a deep heel cup, along with ankle-high shoes for support, will help stabilize your foot

Until trigger points are inactivated, walk or run only on smooth surfaces, start with short distances, and increase mileage gradually. Try rowing, swimming, or bicycling instead.

When sleeping, keep your feet at a 90-degree neutral angle, with the toes neither pointed nor flexed toward the knees. Try putting a pillow against the bottom of your feet to maintain that position.

Keep your lower legs warm and covered. Avoid cold drafts, and use a space heater near your legs if necessary. Protect your feet from cold floors.

If the accelerator pedal in your car is at a steep vertical angle, try putting a wedge on the pedal with the big end at the bottom to reduce the angle of your foot. If it is nearly horizontal, try putting the big end of the wedge at the top. Using cruise control will help. Take breaks every thirty to sixty minutes.

Read "Shin Splints and Tibial Periosteal Stress Syndromes" in chapter 3. Trigger points in the long toe extensors can cause tibial periosteal stress, which is sometimes called "anterior shin splints."

Read "Compartment Syndromes" in chapter 3. If you have a compartment syndrome, *it is important to see a doctor for treatment immediately.*

Self-Help Techniques

Caution: Do not apply pressure to your legs if you have varicose veins in the area to be treated— it could release a clot that could go to your heart or brain! *An acupuncturist or massage therapist should treat your legs, because they can avoid the veins.* You may still do the stretch below.

Applying Pressure

Long Toe Extensors Pressure

Get down on the floor on all fours, and place the tennis ball under the front of your lower leg. Try to bring your lower leg in toward the other leg, so you are getting to the front-outside angle of your lower leg (otherwise you are working on the tibialis anterior). The weight of your leg should give you enough pressure. If you need more or less pressure, shift your weight toward or away from the side you are working on.

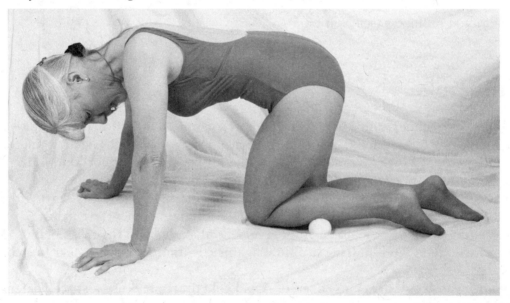

Then lie on your side with the tennis ball under your lower leg, again working toward the front-outside angle of the lower leg (see chapter 18 for the peroneal pressure techniques, but try to work farther forward).

Stretches

The tibialis anterior stretch (see chapter 19) also stretches the long extensors of the toes.

Also See

- Peroneal Muscles (chapter 18)

- Tibialis Anterior (chapter 19)

Conclusion

You may also need to search for trigger points in the peroneal muscles, extensor digitorum brevis, and interossei muscles, since these will also refer pain to the top of the foot, toes, and ankle, and are easily confused with referral from trigger points in the extensor digitorum longus. Also search the extensor hallucis brevis and the tibialis anterior muscles, since trigger point referrals from these muscles are easily confused with those from the extensor hallucis longus.

Chapter 22

Superficial Intrinsic Foot Muscles

The intrinsic muscles of the foot control toe movement. They function as a unit to provide flexibility for shock absorption and balance as well as rigidity and stability for walking.

Because of the deep, aching pain caused by trigger points in these muscles, you may have attempted to get relief by trying many different kinds of shoes and inserts. Inactivating trigger points is crucial to eliminating pain. If you think you have an ankle sprain, but only feel pain in the foot and not the ankle area, it is likely from trigger points in these muscles and not a sprain.

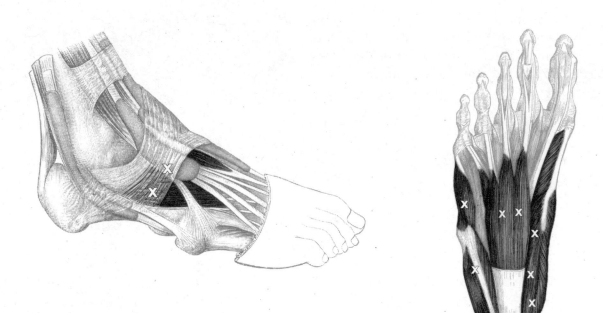

Common Symptoms

- Trigger points refer pain and tenderness within your foot, but not all the way up into your ankle or lower leg.

- You may have deep, aching pain even when not using your feet.

- You probably have a tendency to limp and an inability to walk very far due to pain.

- Orthotics may be uncomfortable if they press against trigger points.

- Tightness and trigger points can lead to plantar fasciitis, especially when combined with tightness in other muscles (see below).

- Trigger points in the extensor digitorum brevis and extensor hallucis brevis muscles refer pain to the top of your foot, but slightly more toward the outside of your foot.

- Trigger points in the abductor hallucis muscle refer pain and tenderness mainly to the inner side of your heel, with some spillover pain on the side above the arch and the backside of your heel. Trigger points in the abductor hallucis muscle can entrap the posterior tibial nerve and its two branches (the medial and lateral plantar nerves) against the medial tarsal bones, possibly causing tarsal tunnel syndrome.

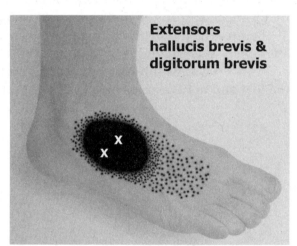

Extensors hallucis brevis & digitorum brevis

- Trigger points in the abductor digiti minimi muscle mainly refer pain to the ball of your foot behind the fifth toe, and possibly back a little farther onto the sole of your foot.

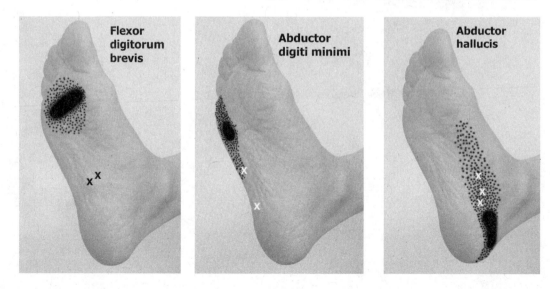

Flexor digitorum brevis

Abductor digiti minimi

Abductor hallucis

- Trigger points in the flexor digitorum brevis muscle refer pain and tenderness to the ball of the foot behind the second, third, and fourth toes, and patients will usually say they have a "sore foot."

Possible Causes and Perpetuators

Injuries or Muscle Abuse

- Wearing shoes that are too tight around the toes and ball of your foot, or inflexible shoes (such as clogs)

- Injuries received by banging or stubbing your toes, or by falling

- Repeatedly using your feet to pull yourself closer to your desk on a rolling chair

- Walking or running on uneven ground or a side-slant

Medical or Structural

- A fracture of the ankle or other bones of the foot, especially if a cast was used

- A longer second toe causing foot rocking can lead to trigger points in the abductor digiti minimi and abductor hallucis muscles

- Foot pronation or supination (standing unevenly on the outside or inside of your feet)

- Hypomobility or hypermobility of the joints of the foot

- Gout (diagnosed with a blood test)

Helpful Hints

Plantar fasciitis is caused by tension overload on the fascial attachment (plantar aponeurosis) on the big bone in the heel, due to tightness in the gastrocnemius (chapter 15), soleus (chapter 16), abductor hallucis, flexor digitorum brevis, and/or abductor digiti minimi muscles. The quadratus plantae (chapter 23) may also be involved. See "Plantar Fasciitis, Heel Pain, and Heel Spurs" in chapter 3 for more information on plantar fasciitis.

If your ankle is hypomobile (doesn't have much movement), see a chiropractor or osteopathic physician to increase mobility. If it is hypermobile (moves too much), orthotics with good arch support and a deep heel cup, along with ankle-high shoes for support, will help stabilize the foot.

Read "Bunions and Hallux Valgus" in chapter 3. Avoid high heels, shoes with narrow toes, and inflexible or slippery soles. Feet get wider and longer with age, so old shoes should be discarded. Pick a shoe with a wide base and cushioning, such as an athletic shoe.

Until trigger points are inactivated, walk or run only on smooth surfaces, start with short distances, and increase mileage gradually. Try rowing, swimming, or bicycling instead.

Self-Help Techniques

Applying Pressure

Superficial Intrinsic Foot Muscles

Sit in a chair and place your foot on top of a golf ball. You may roll it to different spots, holding pressure according to the general guidelines in chapter 7. Be sure to get into the edge of the arch and all the way out to the outside edge of the foot. As tenderness decreases, you can use your forearm to lean on your thigh to add pressure. If you need even more pressure, you can stand with your foot resting on the ball, but *do not shift your weight to that side so that you are actually standing on the ball.*

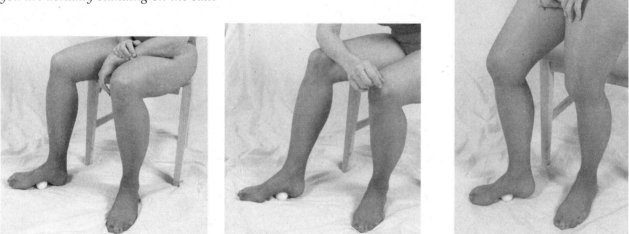

Then put your foot across the opposite thigh and wrap your hands around your foot. Use your thumbs to massage and apply pressure to the inside edge of your arch (where you cannot reach with the golf ball while your foot is on the floor).

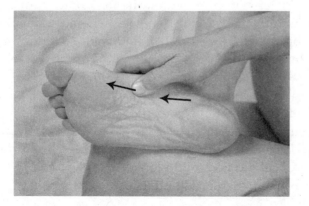

To treat trigger points in the extensors hallucis brevis and digitorum brevis, use your fingers or thumbs on the top of the foot, forward of the outside ankle bone.

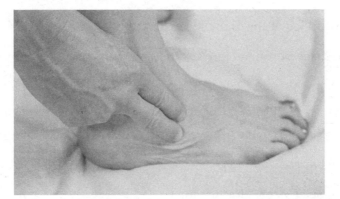

Stretches

Toe Flexors Stretch

Put your foot over the opposite knee, and use the opposite hand to stabilize the ankle. Use the hand on the same side as you are treating to pull up on the toes, until you feel the stretch along the entire foot. Doing this in warm water increases the benefits of the stretch.

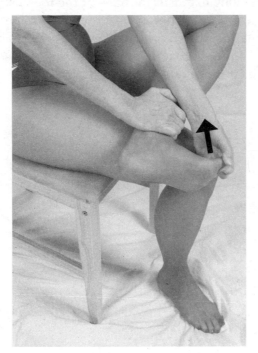

Also See

- Long Extensor Muscles of the Toes: see extensor digitorum longus (chapter 21)

- Peroneal Muscles: see peroneus longus and peroneus brevis (chapter 18)

- Deep Intrinsic Foot Muscles: see adductor hallucis, flexor hallucis brevis, interossei (chapter 23)

- Long Flexor Muscles of the Toes: see flexor digitorum longus (chapter 20)

- Gastrocnemius (chapter 15)

- Soleus/Plantaris: see soleus (chapter 16)

- Deep Intrinsic Foot Muscles: see quadratus plantae (chapter 23)

Conclusion

Search for trigger points in the long extensor muscles of the toes (extensor digitorum longus) and peroneal muscles (peroneus longus and peroneus brevis), since referral patterns are similar to trigger points in the extensor hallucis brevis and extensor digitorum brevis. Also search for trigger points in the deep intrinsic foot muscles (adductor hallucis, interossei) and long flexor muscles of the toes (flexor digitorum longus), since referral patterns are similar to that of trigger points in the flexor digitorum brevis.

Chapter 23

Deep Intrinsic Foot Muscles

Like the superficial intrinsic foot muscles (chapter 22), the deeper muscles move the toes and provide the same functions. The deep muscles probably help the toes adjust to variations in terrain and to dig in more effectively when walking on soft surfaces, such as sand.

Muscular imbalances in the foot, along with misaligned joints, may lead to problems in the knee, hip, pelvis, and spine; therefore, treating trigger points in the feet and resolving the associated perpetuating factors may be crucial to resolving problems in other areas of the body.

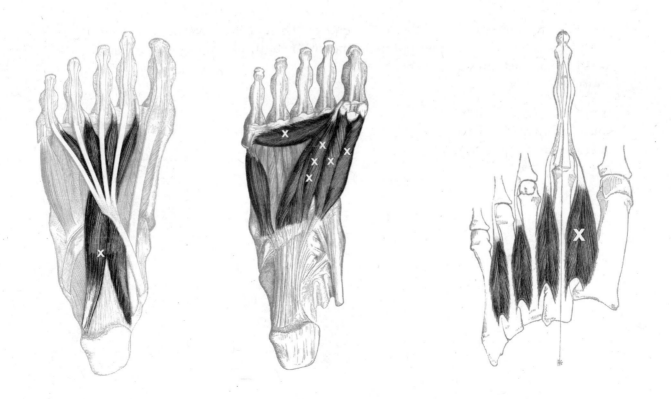

Common Symptoms

- Trigger points in the quadratus plantae muscle refer pain and tenderness to the bottom of the heel.

- Trigger points in the adductor hallucis muscle refer pain to the ball of the foot and are likely to cause a strange, "fluffy" feeling of numbness and a sense of swelling of the skin over the ball of the foot.

- Trigger points in the flexor hallucis brevis muscle refer pain and tenderness to the ball of the foot adjacent to the big toe, and on the outside and top of the big toe, with spill-over pain that may include most of the second toe.

- Trigger points in the interossei muscles refer pain down the top of the toe closest to the affected muscle, and onto the ball of the foot in an area closest to the affected muscle.

- Trigger points in the interosseous muscle between the first and second metatarsals (behind the big and second toes) can cause tingling in the big toe that may also travel into the top of the foot and shin.

- Trigger points in the interossei muscles can cause hammer toes, which may disappear after inactivation of trigger points, particularly in younger people.

- Trigger points in the deep intrinsic foot muscles are usually found in combination with trigger points in other muscles that refer pain to the foot.

- Walking is limited due to pain.

- You may have numbness of the entire end of the foot accompanied by a feeling of swelling, mostly from trigger points in the flexor digiti minimi brevis, flexor hallucis brevis, or adductor hallucis muscles.

- You may have an intolerance to wearing orthotic inserts due to pressure on the trigger points.

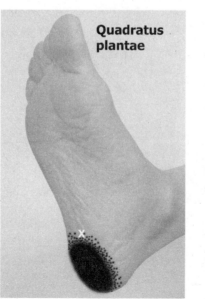

Quadratus plantae

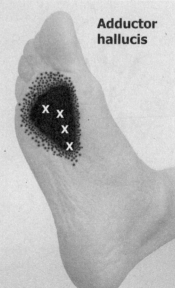

Adductor hallucis

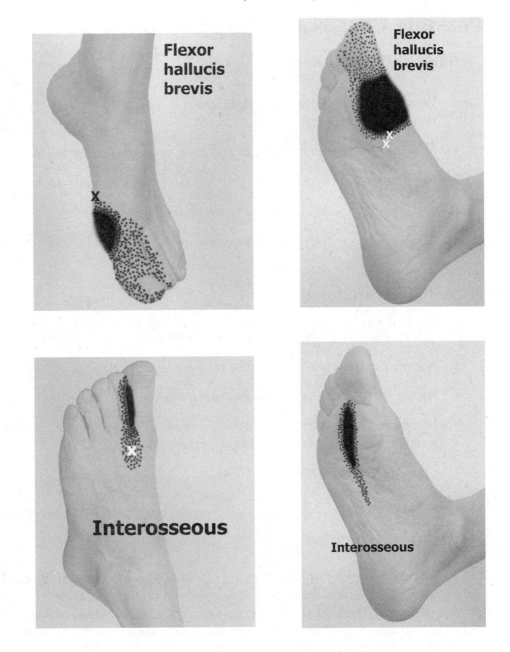

Flexor hallucis brevis

Flexor hallucis brevis

Interosseous

Interosseous

Possible Causes and Perpetuators

Injuries or Muscle Abuse

- Wearing shoes that are too tight around the toes and ball of your foot, or inflexible shoes (such as clogs)

- Injuries received by banging or stubbing your toes, or by falling

- Repeatedly using your feet to pull yourself closer to your desk on a rolling chair

- Walking or running on uneven ground or a side-slant

- Chilling your feet in cold water or wearing wet socks in cold weather

Medical or Structural

- A fracture of the ankle or other bones of the foot, especially if a cast was used

- A longer second toe causing foot rocking

- Foot pronation or supination (standing unevenly on the outside or inside of your feet)

- Hypomobility or hypermobility of the joints of the foot, where there is either not enough movement or too much movement in the joints

- Gout (diagnosed with a blood test)

Helpful Hints

The pain and tenderness from quadratus plantae trigger points can be confused with plantar fasciitis. Plantar fasciitis is caused by tension overload on the fascial attachment (plantar aponeurosis) on the big bone in the heel, due to tightness in the gastrocnemius (chapter 15), soleus (chapter 16), abductor hallucis, flexor digitorum brevis, and/or abductor digiti minimi (chapter 22) muscles. The quadratus plantae (see above) may also be involved. See "Plantar Fasciitis, Heel Pain, and Heel Spurs" in chapter 3 for more information on plantar fasciitis.

If your ankle is hypomobile (doesn't have much movement), see a chiropractor or osteopathic physician to increase mobility. If it is hypermobile (moves too much), orthotics with good arch support and a deep heel cup, along with ankle-high shoes for support, will help stabilize your foot.

Read "Bunions and Hallux Valgus" in chapter 3. Avoid high heels, shoes with narrow toes, and inflexible or slippery soles. Feet get wider and longer with age, so old shoes should be discarded. Pick a shoe with a wide base and cushioning, such as an athletic shoe.

Until trigger points are inactivated, walk or run only on smooth surfaces, start with short distances, and increase mileage gradually. Try rowing, swimming, or bicycling instead.

Self-Help Techniques

You may need to treat the extensor digitorum brevis (chapter 22) and/or extensor digitorum longus (chapter 21) first in order to prevent reactive cramping when you release the deep intrinsic foot muscles.

Applying Pressure

Start with the same pressure techniques as in chapter 22.

Interossei Pressure

Buy an eraser that fits on the end of a pencil. Using the tip of the eraser, press in between the bones of the foot, on both the top and the bottom. You may hold pressure, but also move the eraser back and forth in the groove in between the long bones of the foot.

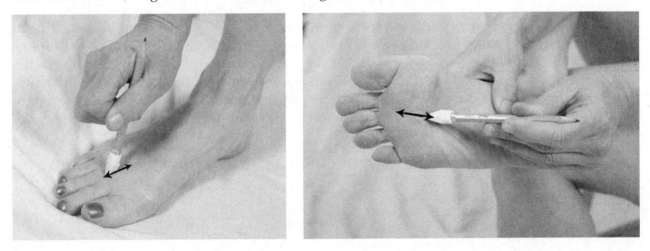

Stretches

The stretches and exercises are the same as in chapter 22.

Also See

- Soleus/Plantaris: see soleus (chapter 16)

- Gastrocnemius (chapter 15)

- Long Flexor Muscles of the Toes (chapter 20)

- Superficial Intrinsic Foot Muscles: see flexor digitorum brevis, abductor hallucis (chapter 22)

- Tibialis Anterior (chapter 19)

- Long Extensor Muscles of the Toes: see extensor hallucis longus (chapter 21)

Conclusion

Also search for trigger points in the gastrocnemius, soleus, flexor digitorum longus, and abductor hallucis muscles, since they can have referral patterns somewhat similar to that of the quadratus plantae. Search the gastrocnemius, flexor digitiorum longus, and flexor digitorum brevis muscles, since referral patterns from those trigger points can be confused with those of the adductor hallucis. Search the tibialis anterior, extensor hallucis longus, and flexor hallucis longus muscles, since those trigger points could be confused with referral patterns for the flexor hallucis brevis muscle.

Resources

New Harbinger Publications. New Harbinger publishes books on a variety of self-help topics that you may find helpful. 800-748-6273. newharbinger.com.

The Pressure Positive Company. This company sells self-pressure devices and massage tools. Their website has an information center with articles and links to other helpful sites. 800-603-5107. pressurepositive.com.

Superfeet. This company sells noncorrective footbeds, and their website can help you locate a dealer who can make Superfeet custom footbeds for you. 800-634-6618. superfeet.com.

TriggerPointRelief.com. Author's website with additional resources, articles, and links to helpful sites.

References

Audette, J. F., F. Wang, and H. Smith. 2004. Bilateral activation of motor unit potentials with unilateral needle stimulation of active myofascial trigger points. *American Journal of Physical Medicine and Rehabilitation* 83(5):368–74.

Balch, J. F., and P. A. Balch. 2000. *Prescription for Nutritional Healing: A Practical A–Z Reference to Drug-Free Remedies Using Vitamins, Minerals, Herbs, and Food Supplements.* New York: Avery.

Borg-Stein, J., and D. G. Simons. 2002. Myofascial pain. *Archives of Physical Medicine and Rehabilitation* 83(Suppl 1):S40–47.

Chen Q., S. Bensamoun, J. R. Basford, J. M. Thompson, and K. N. An. 2007. Identification of myofascial taut bands with magnetic resonance elastography. *Archives of Physical Medicine and Rehabilitation* 88:1658–1661.

Edwards, J., and N. Knowles. 2003. Superficial dry needling and active stretching in the treatment of myofascial pain: A randomised controlled trial. *Acupuncture in Medicine* 21(3):80–86.

Hinkers, M. 2009. Diabetes: Taking steps to prevent amputation. *Lower Extremity Review* 1(2):33–40.

Issbener, U., P. Reeh, and K. Steen. 1996. Pain due to tissue acidosis: A mechanism for inflammatory and ischemic myalgia? *Neuroscience Letters* 208 (1996):191–194.

Kuan, T. 2009. Current studies on myofascial pain syndrome. *Current Pain and Headache Reports* 13:365–369.

Latremoliere, A., and C. J. Woolf. 2009. Central sensitization: A generator of pain hypersensitivity by central neural plasticity. *The Journal of Pain* 10(9):895–926.

Li, J. , and C. Muehleman. 2007. Anatomic relationship of heel spur to surrounding soft tissues: Greater variability than previously reported. *Clinical Anatomy* 20:950–955.

Marcus, D. A., L. Scharff, S. Mercer, and D. C. Turk. 1999. Musculoskeletal abnormalities in chronic headache: A controlled comparison of headache diagnostic groups. *Headache: The Journal of Head and Face Pain* 39(1):21–27.

Murphy, L., T. Z. Schwartz, C. G. Helmick, J. B. Renner, G. Tudor, G. Koch, A. Dragomir, W. D. Kalsbeek, G. Luta, and J. M. Jordan. 2008. Lifetime risk of symptomatic knee osteoarthritis. *Arthritis and Rheumatism* 59(9):1207–1213.

Niddam, D. M. 2009. Brain manifestation and modulation of pain from myofascial trigger points. *Current Pain and Headache Reports* 13:370–375.

Partanen, J., T. A. Ojala, and J. P. A. Arokoski. 2009. Myofascial syndrome and pain: A neurophysiologic approach. *Pathophysiology*, doi:10.10266/j.pathophus.2009.05.001.

Shah, J. P., J. V. Danoff, M. J. Desai, S. Parikh, L. Y. Nakamura, T. M. Phillips, and L. H. Gerber. 2008. Biochemicals associated with pain and inflammation are elevated in sites near to and remote from active myofascial trigger points. *Archives of Physical Medicine and Rehabilitation* 89:16–23.

Simons, D. G. 2003. Enigmatic trigger points often cause enigmatic musculoskeletal pain. Presentation at the STAR Symposium, Columbus, Ohio, May 22. Available at http://ergonomics.osu.edu/pdfs/2003%20STAR%20Symposium/Simons%20Trigger.pdf.

———. 2004. Review of enigmatic MTrPs as a common cause of enigmatic musculoskeletal pain and dysfunction. *Journal of Electromyography and Kinesiology* 14(1):95–107.

Simons, D. G., J. G. Travell, and L. S. Simons. 1999. *Myofascial Pain and Dysfunction: The Trigger Point Manual.* Vol. 1, *The Upper Extremities,* 2nd ed. Baltimore, MD: Lippincott Williams & Wilkins.

Travell, J. G., and D. G. Simons. 1983. *Myofascial Pain and Dysfunction: The Trigger Point Manual.* Baltimore, MD: Lippincott Williams & Wilkins.

———. 1992. *Myofascial Pain and Dysfunction: The Trigger Point Manual.* Vol. 2, *The Lower Extremities.* Baltimore, MD: Lippincott Williams & Wilkins.

Wickstrom, E., and M. Cordova. 2009. Ankle balance training targets recurrent injury. *Lower Extremity Review* 1(3):51–54.

Index

Valerie DeLaune, L.Ac., is a licensed acupuncturist and certified neuromuscular therapist who teaches trigger point workshops nationally. She holds a master's degree in acupuncture from the Northwest Institute of Acupuncture and Oriental Medicine, a bachelor of science degree from the University of Washington, and professional certificates from the Heartwood Institute and the Brenneke School of Massage. DeLaune is author of many books and articles on trigger points and acupuncture. She currently resides in Alaska. www.triggerpointrelief.com

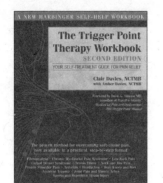
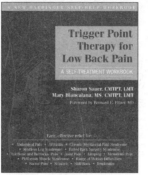
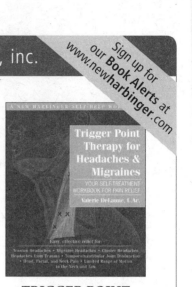
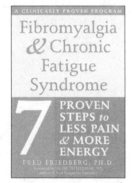
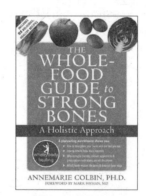
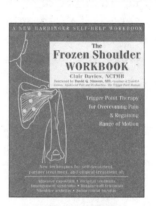